THERAPEUTIC STRETCHING

Log on to www.therapeuticstretch.com

Dedicated, as always, to Tsafi, Mattan, Guy and Pinuki

Content Strategist: Alison Taylor
Content Development Specialist: Catherine Jackson
Project Manager: Kiruthiga Kasthuriswamy/Beula Christopher
Photographers, Chapter 13: David Hughes and Sascha Panknin
Designer/Design Direction: Miles Hitchen
Illustration Manager: Jennifer Rose
Illustrator: Ethan Danielson

THERAPEUTIC STRETCHING

Towards a functional approach

Eyal Lederman DO, PhD

Director, Centre for Professional Development
in Manual and Physical Therapies;
Senior Lecturer, University College London (UCL),
London, UK.

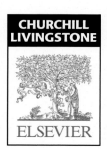

Edinburgh London New York Oxford Philadelphia St Louis Sydney Toronto 2014

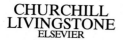

ISBN: 978-0-7020-4318-5

British Library Cataloguing in Publication Data
A catalogue record for this book is available from the British Library

Library of Congress Cataloging in Publication Data
A catalog record for this book is available from the Library of Congress

Notices

Knowledge and best practice in this field are constantly changing. As new research and experience broaden our understanding, changes in research methods, professional practices, or medical treatment may become necessary.

Practitioners and researchers must always rely on their own experience and knowledge in evaluating and using any information, methods, compounds, or experiments described herein. In using such information or methods they should be mindful of their own safety and the safety of others, including parties for whom they have a professional responsibility.

With respect to any drug or pharmaceutical products identified, readers are advised to check the most current information provided (i) on procedures featured or (ii) by the manufacturer of each product to be administered, to verify the recommended dose or formula, the method and duration of administration, and contraindications. It is the responsibility of practitioners, relying on their own experience and knowledge of their patients, to make diagnoses, to determine dosages and the best treatment for each individual patient, and to take all appropriate safety precautions.

To the fullest extent of the law, neither the Publisher nor the authors, contributors, or editors, assume any liability for any injury and/or damage to persons or property as a matter of products liability, negligence or otherwise, or from any use or operation of any methods, products, instructions, or ideas contained in the material herein.

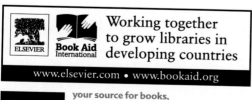

www.elsevier.com • www.bookaid.org

your source for books,
journals and multimedia
in the health sciences
www.elsevierhealth.com

The
publisher's
policy is to use
**paper manufactured
from sustainable forests**

Printed in China

Contents

Preface

Stretching has many uses and forms and is one of the principal tools used in physical therapies. However, in the last decade and a half the therapeutic value of stretching has been eroded by research. These findings leave us with a difficult choice: to ignore them and become clinically irrelevant, or to progress by accepting and incorporating them into our practice. Incorporating these findings means that we have to transform our thinking and the way we apply stretching clinically. This is not a simple task; in particular, as stretching techniques have remained virtually unchanged for decades, or even centuries.

This book is all about the direction and changes that we may need to consider, and how to apply them clinically. In particular, it explores the use of stretching in conditions in which individuals experience a loss in range of movement (ROM).

The book starts by looking at the difference between therapeutic and recreational stretching; whether stretching is a physiological necessity; and the classification of stretching approaches (Ch. 1). This is followed by exploring what constitutes ROM and defining normal and dysfunctional ROM (Ch. 2). From there the book explores the processes associated with ROM loss and recovery, focusing on adaptive processes. Chapters 5–7 explore what makes stretching effective, identifying behaviour as one of the main driving forces for adaptive changes. The motor control component of ROM, and how it is influenced by different stretching methods, is discussed in Chapter 8. The experience of pain, sensitization and pain tolerance in relation to stretching and ROM recovery are discussed in Chapters 9 and 10. In Chapter 11 the psychological considerations in ROM management are addressed, and Chapter 12 integrates all the information from previous chapters and presents a functional approach in therapeutic stretching. This approach uses the individual's unique movement repertoire to help them regain functionality. A demonstration of this approach is found in Chapter 13 and on the accompanying website. A grand summary of the book is found in Chapter 14.

Interestingly, the message from the sciences is that we should be moving towards a bio-psycho-behavioural-social approach for ROM rehabilitation; away from traditional stretching models that focus on biomechanics and structure. The premise here is that ROM recovery is a multidimensional process intrinsic to the individual but also highly influenced by their environment. The locus of recovery is intrinsic to the patient, not external in the "therapist's hands". As such, the role of the therapist needs to be reconsidered: from a provider of cure to a facilitator of recovery; providing support, direction, management and assistance. It is an approach that promotes self-care.

To write this book I have used several sources: studies in the areas of biomechanics, biomedicine and health studies, motor control, psychology, cognition and behaviour, and my own research. Yet, I still found that, despite this vast volume of published research, many theoretical and practical questions about stretching remain unanswered. A pure science-based book about stretching was therefore not the solution. As a consequence, I have committed the sin of adding my experiences from physical therapy teaching and supervising clinicians, yoga instruction, clinical work that spans 26 years and a dose of what seems (to me) like common sense.

This book is suitable for all manual and physical therapists, sports and personal trainers, athletes who require special movement ranges and individuals who would like to recover or improve their range and ease of movement. I hope that this book will present an insight into the fascinating world of stretching and provide you and your patients with an effective therapeutic approach.

Dr. Eyal Lederman
London 2013
Information on courses: www.cpdo.net

THE WEBSITE

Besides the wealth of information found within *Therapeutic Stretching: Towards a Functional Approach*, the Publishers have created a unique website – www.therapeuticstretch.com – to accompany the volume. This site contains a selection of video clips which have been specially prepared to allow the reader to practice the techniques described in the volume.

To access the site, go to www.therapeuticstretch.com and follow the simple log-on instructions shown.

CHAPTER 1

Introduction to Therapeutic and Functional Stretching

Stiffness and restricted range of movement (ROM) are the most common clinical presentations second to pain. This book is for all therapists and individuals who would like to help others or themselves to recover or improve their ease and ROM. The book aims to provide the know-how to achieve this therapeutic goal with maximum effect.

WHAT IS STRETCHING?

For the purpose of this book stretching is defined as *the behaviour a person adopts to recover, increase or maintain their range of movement*. This behaviour includes passive and active stretching, which can be in the form of exercise or with the assistance of another person (therapist/trainer). Stretching therefore is the means by which the ROM can be increased, but it is not the only one. There are several ways to achieve ROM improvements depending on the processes associated with the loss of ROM. *ROM rehabilitation* is perhaps a more suitable term to describe the therapeutic method used to recover/improve movement range. *ROM challenge* is the term given to all the different methods and techniques that are used to achieve this movement goal (Fig. 1.1).

THERAPEUTIC, SPORTS AND RECREATIONAL STRETCHING

Stretching behaviour can be observed in many spheres of human activity. It is often used in sports training as a warm-up, for prevention of injury and to improve sports performance. It is widely used by specialist groups such as athletes and yoga practitioners to develop the high level of flexibility required for performance/practice. Stretching is also used recreationally for general flexibility, enjoyment and self-awareness, as part of spiritual development, and for supporting health and well-being (e.g. yoga, Pilates and t'ai chi). Therapeutic

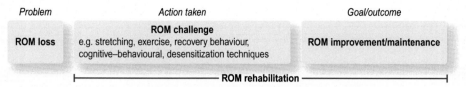

FIGURE 1.1 Terminology used in therapeutic stretching. ROM, range of movement.

stretching is used predominantly to help individuals to regain functionality that has been affected by ROM losses, and occasionally to alleviate pain (Fig. 1.2).

Therapeutic stretching, recreational stretching and sports stretching depend on the same biological–physiological processes to promote ROM changes. The differences are in their overall goals (recover ROM or feel great) and the context in which the ROM challenges are applied (in clinic or in a yoga class). The definition of stretching given above can also be used to define ROM rehabilitation or therapeutic stretching.

This book will focus on the therapeutic use of stretching and ROM rehabilitation. However, many of the principles discussed here can be applied to recreational and athletic stretching.

Is stretching essential for normalization of ROM?

It seems that only humans do it; that is, regular, systematic stretching. There is a shared animal and human behaviour of "having a stretch" and yawning

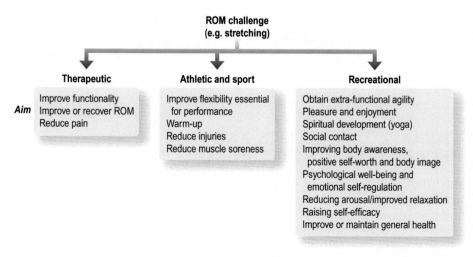

FIGURE 1.2 Categories of stretching and their aims. Whether these aims are realistic or achievable will be discussed in the book. ROM, range of movement.

called *pandiculation*. It is often a combination of elongating, shortening and stiffening of muscles throughout the body. Pandiculation tends to occur more frequently in the morning and evening and is associated with waking, fatigue and drowsiness.[1] Erroneously, it is assumed that animals use pandiculation as a form of stretch. This behaviour is too short in duration, too infrequent and too specific to a particular pattern to account for general agility. It has been proposed that pandiculation may provide psychological and physiological benefits other than flexibility.[1,2]

Among humans, only relatively few individuals stretch regularly. Those who stretch tend to focus on particular parts of the body. For example, rarely is the little finger stretched into extension or the forearm into full pronation–supination. So what happens to the majority who do not stretch? Do they gradually stiffen into a solid unyielding dysfunctional mass? And what happens to the parts that we never stretch? Do they stand out as being stiff/range-restricted?

It seems that going about our daily activities provides sufficient challenges to maintain functional ranges; otherwise, we would all suffer from some catastrophic stiffening fate. This suggests that stretching is not a biological–physiological necessity but perhaps a socio-cultural construct. We stretch because it provides special flexibility, it is fashionable and enjoyable (for some), and some believe that it is essential for maintenance of healthy posture and movement. There may be other benefits to recreational stretching such as improving body awareness, positive self-worth and body image, psychological well-being, reduced arousal/improved relaxation, emotional self-regulation and raising self-efficacy.

However, the most important message from the discussion so far is that *functional movement, the natural movement repertoire of the individual*, is sufficient to maintain the normal ROM. It suggests that ROM rehabilitation, in its most basic form, should put an emphasis on return to pre-injury activities, whenever possible.

Is stretching useful therapeutically?

Recovering ROM becomes important when a person is unable to perform normal daily activities, often as a result of some pathological process that results in range limitation. So there is an obvious need for ROM rehabilitation, but the question is which ROM challenges are most effective?

It has been assumed for a long time that traditional stretching approaches can provide effective ROM challenges. This assumption was supported by numerous studies demonstrating that in healthy young individuals regular stretching results in ROM improvements. Since the biological processes for

ROM improvements are similar to those for recovery, the logical conclusion was that stretching is clinically useful. However, only in the last decade has the use of stretching been explored clinically, as a treatment for contractures after joint surgery, neurological conditions and immobilization. The outcome of these studies was summarized in 2010 in a systematic review (35 studies with a total of 1391 subjects).[3] It was found that in the short term stretching provides a 3° improvement, a 1° improvement in the medium term and no influence in the long term (up to 7 months). These findings were similar to all stretching approaches, active or passive. Let us assume for the sake of discussion that these reviewers underestimated the effects of stretching. Stretching will still be clinically irrelevant even if these results are doubled (6° and 2°) or tripled (9° and 3°).[4] Such modest changes would be meaningless as far as functional activities are concerned;[5] most patients (in my experience) would consider this outcome a treatment failure.

The erosion of belief in the usefulness of stretching is also seen in other areas. Stretching as a warm-up before and after exercising has failed to show any benefit for alleviating muscle soreness. It provides no protection against sports injuries and vigorous stretching before an event may even reduce sports performance.[6-16] It was demonstrated that strength performance can be reduced by 4.5–28%, irrespective of the stretching technique used.[17,18]

One reason that stretching was not shown to be useful in all these areas may go back to biological necessity. If it was beneficial we would expect Nature to have "factored-in" stretching as part of animal behaviour, in particular if it improved performance. Yet, with the exception of humans, no animal performs any pre-exertion activities that resemble a stretch warm-up. Lions do not limber up with a stretch before they chase their prey, and reciprocally the prey does not halt the chase for the lack of a stretch. The stretch warm-up in humans seems to be largely ceremonial. A person would stretch in the park before a jog but would not consider stretching to be important for sprinting after a bus. A person may stretch before lifting weights in the gym but a builder is unlikely to stretch, although they may be lifting and carrying throughout the day. The point made here is that we have evolved to perform maximally, instantly and without the need to limber up with stretching. There seems to be no biological advantage in stretching nor is it physiologically essential.

The ineffectiveness of stretching leaves us with the clinical conundrum of how to recover ROM losses. We do know that most of the time people do recover their ROM losses after conditions such as immobilization, surgery, disuse and even frozen shoulder. If they do not do this by stretching, some other phenomenon must account for the recovery; but what is it and can it guide us to a more effective ROM rehabilitation?

TOWARDS A FUNCTIONAL–BEHAVIOURAL APPROACH

The place to start exploring the solution to ROM rehabilitation is the natural *recovery behaviour* seen after an injury or immobility. There seems to be a universal behaviour in which the individual will attempt to perform the affected movement in a guarded progressive manner. A person who has limited reaching ROM will attempt that same movement, gradually increasing the range of reaching, forces used to lift or speed of that particular movement. Through such behavioural experiences the individual learns that taking certain actions will eventually help them to achieve their movement goals. So the recovery of ROM is driven by the individual's actions or behaviour.

Imagine if somehow "the essence" of the recovery behaviour could be extracted and provided to patients who are not improving naturally. The recovery behaviour contains three identifiable traits that are beneficial for improving ROM. The movement closely resembles the affected daily functional tasks and it is repeated many times throughout the day. The recovery behaviour also contains movements that are progressively amplified to provide increasing physical demands on the body. These components of the recovery behaviour are similar to the *specificity*, *overloading* and *repetition* principles used to optimize sports performance. Thus, a ROM rehabilitation programme can be constructed by simply amplifying these three traits. The management for a person with a shoulder problem who cannot reach overhead is to attempt this particular movement (specificity; Ch. 5), trying to reach further overhead (overloading; Ch. 6), many times during the day (repetition; Ch. 7). It is basically about performing functional activities with an emphasis on end-ranges. This form of ROM rehabilitation is termed *managed recovery behaviour*.

Managed recovery behaviour assumes that the patient is able to self-care and can maintain a rehabilitation programme. However, some patients may need assistance, a "helping hand" from others. In the assisted programme the essence of the recovery behaviour is still the guiding model. The therapist helps the patient to reach the end-ranges. In these positions the patient attempts to perform a variety of daily movements. For example, in shoulder contractures, the therapist helps the patient to attain a comfortable flexion position. At this angle, the patient is instructed to imagine and perform a functional activity, such as painting the ceiling or waving a flag.

The therapist-assisted form of ROM rehabilitation is termed, here, *functional stretching* (Fig. 1.3). The term functional stretching is used solely for its simplicity. Most practitioners, and more importantly patients, can understand its meaning and aims. This approach is discussed in greater detail in Chapter 12, and presented in Chapter 13 and the accompanying video.

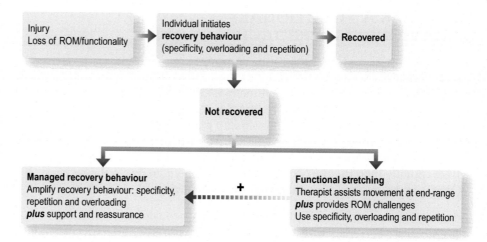

FIGURE 1.3 Using elements from the recovery behaviour as a basis for a functional range of movement (ROM) rehabilitation (see expansion of this chart in Ch. 12).

ROM challenges and management that are modelled on the recovery behaviour are termed, here, *functional challenges* or *functional ROM rehabilitation*. The reason for choosing one form of management over another depends on patient-related factors (Fig. 1.3). A managed approach could be beneficial for patients who may need psychological/emotional support in their journey of recovery, or simply need help in identifying suitable daily challenges and organizing/scheduling their rehabilitation programme. An assisted approach is often used when the patient is unable to self-provide/fulfil the recovery behaviour because of physical incapacity or pain (see Ch. 12).

Advantages of functional challenges

There are several advantages to functional ROM rehabilitation. Functional challenges are essentially "exaggeration" of the individual's normal daily movements. Hence, the patient uses movement patterns they are familiar with; they do not have to learn anything new. Functional challenges can be practised anywhere and anytime, thereby reducing the need for special equipment or set-aside time for training. There is also a strong motivational factor in functional challenges. There is a clear resemblance between the movement used in the clinical session and the patient's functionality goals and hopes; imagine rehabilitating a person who is unable to play tennis by using tennis as a ROM challenge.

A functional approach promotes individualization of the management. It is tailored to the patient's movement repertoire, needs and therapeutic goals. These factors could help to increase compliance and adherence to the rehabilitation programme, which is particularly important as most ROM losses are chronic conditions in which self-care is essential for success. There is a strong indication from the sciences that such inclusive management could provide clinical solutions where traditional stretching methods may have failed (see Chapters 2–14).

TOWARDS A PROCESS APPROACH

ROM loss and recovery is a multidimensional process intrinsic to the individual but also highly influenced by their environment. It is often a complex mixture of processes that occur within biological, neurological and psychological dimensions (Fig. 1.4).

The tissue dimension is mostly associated with processes such as repair and biomechanical/morphological adaptation of local tissues and local fluid dynamics (lymph, blood). The neurological dimension is mostly associated with motor control and nociceptive processes such as sensitization. The psychological dimension is associated with psychological, cognitive, behavioural, pain experience and psychophysiological processes. These dimensions and related processes are open systems: processes often span several dimensions,

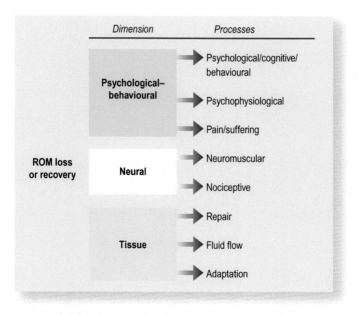

FIGURE 1.4 The dimensional model. Range of movement (ROM) loss but also recovery is associated with dimension specific processes.

but tend to be prominent in particular ones depending on the presenting condition. (For full discussion of the dimensional model, see Lederman.[19])

The complex interaction of processes and dimensions can be illustrated by contractures after immobilization. ROM losses are due to tissue shortening and adhesions, processes that occur within the *tissue dimension* (Ch. 4). Immobilization is also associated with an adaptive dysfunctional motor control that limits the ability to perform the *active* ROM, a process that occurs in the *neurological dimension* (Chs 4 and 8). The patient's will and level of commitment, psychological distress and pain/movement-related fears may affect their recovery behaviour and consequently their ROM improvements. These processes and their management are occurring within the *psychological– behavioural dimension* (Ch. 11).

Processes underpinning ROM recovery

The recovery from any condition is associated with three basic recuperative processes: repair, adaptation and/or modulation of symptoms (Fig. 1.5). The success of ROM rehabilitation depends on engaging these intrinsic processes.

Repair is a process in which the body restores the functional and structural integrity of damaged tissues. During the period of repair ROM can be affected by various processes that include pain, swelling, protective motor responses

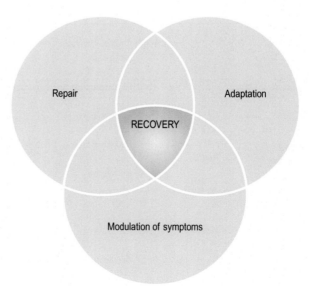

FIGURE 1.5 Recovery from any condition is dependent on repair, adaptation and modulation of symptoms (symptomatic relief). The success of ROM rehabilitation is dependent on these intrinsic recuperative processes.

and movement-related anxieties (Chs 9 and 11). In acute injuries, these ROM losses tend to recover along with the resolution of repair. However, long-term loss and recovery of ROM after an injury is more often associated with adaptation processes.

Adaptation is an alteration in the physiological, biomechanical, morphological and psychological–behavioural characteristics of the body/individual in response to a change in their physical and social environment. ROM recovery is often the consequence of adaptation in several of these processes and dimensions (Ch. 4).

Often ROM losses are associated with the experience of pain, discomfort and stiffness. Hence, some ROM improvement can be down to symptomatic relief. This can come about by various processes: resolution of repair, adaption within the nociceptive system, such as sensitization and de-sensitization (Ch. 9), and "psychological adaptation", such as pain tolerance (Chs 9 and 10). Symptomatic relief can also be homeostatic in nature; a brief response to stimulation and a return to the symptomatic default. This transient response can explain some of the immediate ROM changes observed following some forms of physical therapy (Ch. 9).

A process approach acknowledges the multidimensional processes that underlie ROM loss and recovery and aims to co-create, with the patient, environments that support the recovery processes. It steers away from the traditional orthopaedic–structural models prevalent in physical therapies; models that promote the belief that recovery can be achieved by correcting, balancing and adjusting the body according to a mechanical–structural ideal.[20,21] The functional model of ROM rehabilitation promoted in this book is derived from a process approach.

CLASSIFICATION OF STRETCHING

A functional approach is also the point from which we can classify stretching techniques. As discussed above, recovery behaviour usually consists of functional movement patterns. So the ROM challenges can either resemble or be unlike functional movement (Fig. 1.6). Techniques or movement patterns that resemble the normal daily activities of the individual are called *functional challenges*. ROM challenges that use movement patterns that are outside the individual's repertoire or experience are called *extra-functional challenges*. Lying on the floor and performing straight leg raises to stretch the hamstring is an example of an extra-functional challenge. Most traditional stretching techniques fall within the extra-functional category. They include techniques such as static and dynamic stretching, proprioceptive neuromuscular facilitation (PNF), muscle energy techniques (METs) and ballistic stretching.

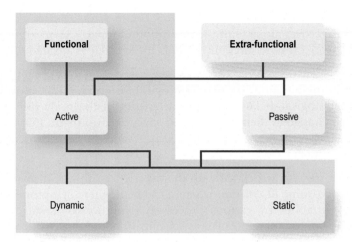

FIGURE 1.6 The classification of range of movement challenges.

Generally, all functional challenges are active. This is because there is no passive movement in the functional repertoire of humans (except short phases during some active movements; see Ch. 2). Extra-functional ROM challenges can be either passive or active, and sometimes they are a mixture of both. Sitting on the floor and forcefully pulling on the foot to stretch the calf muscle is an example of an extra-functional passive approach. A standing calf muscle stretch is an example of an extra-functional active approach. METs and PNF are extra-functional approaches that mix passive and active challenges (Fig. 1.7).

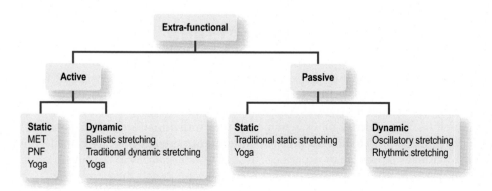

FIGURE 1.7 Classification of extra-functional stretching approaches into active or passive and static or dynamic. Disciplines such as yoga can be both active and passive. MET, muscle energy technique; PNF, proprioceptive neuromuscular facilitation.

Finally, the last subdivision is whether a challenge is dynamic (with movement) or static (no movement). Functional challenges can be either dynamic or static, depending on the task. For example, reaching with the arm to a demanding overhead position is a dynamic functional challenge, whereas maintaining that position is a static functional challenge. Ballistic stretching is an example of a dynamic extra-functional challenge. All techniques in which the therapist stretches and holds the patient at the end-range position can be considered to be static extra-functional challenges.

Throughout the book this classification will be used to discuss stretching and ROM rehabilitation. The term *traditional stretching* refers to all extra-functional challenges.

What about traditional forms of stretching?

All forms of stretching activate some of the intrinsic processes associated with ROM recovery. However, functional challenges optimally engage all traits associated with the recovery behaviour. So there are important therapeutic advantages in using a functional ROM rehabilitation over traditional stretching approaches (see further discussion throughout the book, and in particular Ch. 12). This does not mean that traditional forms of stretching should be given up; we just need to do a lot more of the one (functional) than the other (traditional). This is what this book is all about.

SUMMARY

- ROM rehabilitation is the therapeutic process used to recover or improve movement range
- ROM challenges are the different techniques and methods used to achieve ROM change
- The natural recovery behaviour of an individual after an injury or immobilization is the most widely used ROM challenge
- Recovery behaviour contains three traits that are important for ROM recovery: specificity, repetition and overloading
- Specificity is how closely the ROM challenge resembles the affected functional movement. Repetition is the overall exposure to the challenge, and overloading is the progressive increase in physical demands on the affected movement
- Repair, adaptation and mechanisms associated with symptomatic relief are the processes that underpin ROM recovery
- Recovery processes occur in the tissue, neurological and psychological–behavioural dimensions

- Understanding the processes and dimensions associated with the ROM loss is important for developing and individualizing the rehabilitation programme
- ROM challenges can be either functional or extra-functional. Functional challenges are active approaches that resemble normal movement patterns
- Movements that are dissimilar to daily patterns are termed extra-functional challenges
- Managed recovery behaviour is a functional approach. It is where the therapist helps the patient to develop a self-care daily programme using the specificity, repetition and overloading principles
- Functional stretching is a therapist-assisted functional challenge. It is used when the patient is unable to execute the recovery behaviour
- Many of the traditional stretching methods are extra-functional challenges
- This book focuses on functional approaches in ROM rehabilitation. They include managed recovery behaviour, a self-help approach and functional stretching – a therapist-assisted functional rehabilitation

REFERENCES

1. Bertolucci LF. Pandiculation: nature's way of maintaining the functional integrity of the myofascial system? J Bodyw Mov Ther 2011;15(3):268–80.
2. Campbell MW, de Waal FBM. Ingroup–outgroup bias in contagious yawning by chimpanzees supports link to empathy. PLoS ONE 2011;6(4):e182–3.
3. Katalinic OM, Harvey LA, Herbert RD, et al. Stretch for the treatment and prevention of contractures. Cochrane Database Syst Rev 2010;8(9):CD007455.
4. Macedo LG, Magee DJ. Differences in range of motion between dominant and nondominant sides of upper and lower extremities. J Manipulative Physiol Ther 2008;31(8):577–82.
5. Doege TC, Houston TP. Guide to the evaluation of permanent impairment. 4th ed. Chicago: American Medical Association; 1995.
6. Behm DG, Button DC, Butt JC. Factors affecting force loss with prolonged stretching. Appl Physiol 2001;26(3):261–72.
7. Behm DG. Effect of acute static stretching on force, balance, reaction time, and movement time. Med Sci Sports Exerc 2004;36:1397–402.
8. Brushøj C, Larsen K, Albrecht-Beste E, et al. Prevention of overuse injuries by a concurrent exercise program in subjects exposed to an increase in training load: a randomized controlled trial of 1020 army recruits. Am J Sports Med 2008;36(4):663–70.
9. Witvrouw E, Mahieu N, Danneels L, et al. Stretching and injury prevention: an obscure relationship. Sports Med 2004;34:7443–9.
10. Gremion G. Is stretching for sports performance still useful? A review of the literature. Rev Med Suisse 2005;1(28):1830–4.
11. Andersen JC. Stretching before and after exercise: effect on muscle soreness and injury risk. J Athl Train 2005;40(3):218–20.
12. Shrier I. Does stretching improve performance? A systematic and critical review of the literature. Clin J Sport Med 2004;14(5):267–73.
13. Herbert RD, de Noronha M. Stretching to prevent or reduce muscle soreness after exercise. Cochrane Database Syst Rev 2011;7:CD004577.
14. Ingraham SJ. The role of flexibility in injury prevention and athletic performance: have we stretched the truth? Minn Med 2003;86(5):58–61.

15. Simic L, Sarabon N, Markovic G. Does pre-exercise static stretching inhibit maximal muscular performance? A meta-analytical review. Scand J Med Sci Sports 2012; Feb 8 [Epub ahead of print].

16. Kay AD, Blazevich AJ. Effect of acute static stretch on maximal muscle performance: a systematic review. Med Sci Sports Exerc 2012;44(1):154–64.

17. Young WB, Behm DG. Should static stretching be used during a warm-up for strength and power activities? Strength Cond J 2002;24:33–7.

18. Rubini EC, Costa AL, Gomes PS. The effects of stretching on strength performance. Sports Med 2007;37:213–24.

19. Lederman E. The science and practice of manual therapy. 2nd ed. Edinburgh: Churchill Livingstone; 2005.

20. Lederman E. The fall of the postural–structural–biomechanical model in manual and physical therapies: exemplified by lower back pain. J Bodyw Mov Ther 2011;15(2):131–8.

21. Lederman E. Re: The fall of the postural–structural–biomechanical model in manual therapy: exemplified by lower back pain. A response to reviewers and further thoughts. J Bodyw Mov Ther 2011;15(3):257–8.

CHAPTER 2

Functional and Dysfunctional ROM

In setting out to rehabilitate range of movement (ROM) the first task is to establish what is normal ROM and what is abnormal ROM; and this task is not as simple as it seems. Take two asymptomatic individuals and ask them to bend forwards to touch their toes. One will just about reach their knees while the other will place their hands flat on the floor. Which of these individuals has a normal ROM and which a pathological ROM, the stiffer individual or the hyperflexible individual? Does it matter if the stiffer person cannot reach their toes?

This chapter explores what constitutes ROM, in particular:

- Where is the end-range?
- What are active and passive ranges?
- What is normal ROM?
- When is ROM dysfunctional?
- When is ROM considered to be normalized?

ROM INGREDIENTS

ROM is composed of active and passive movement components. The active ROM is generated by voluntary muscle activation. The passive ROM is the extent to which a joint or a limb can be moved in the absence of voluntary contraction (Fig. 2.1).

Daily activities are mostly voluntary and are therefore performed within the active ROM.[1-5] This, as will be discussed later, has important implications for ROM rehabilitation (Ch. 8). Passive ROMs often constitute a smaller proportion of functional activities. For example, during the terminal phase of walking the ankle is "passively" dorsiflexed by the forward shift of the body over the extended leg. However, such movements are not fully passive. They are often controlled by eccentric activity in the antagonistic muscles. Passive ranges are also observed in particular postures or at rest: passive ankle dorsiflexion during

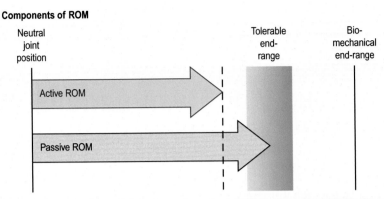

FIGURE 2.1 Normal active–passive range of movement (ROM). The active ROM is the extent to which a person can voluntarily move a joint or limb. The passive ROM is the extent to which a joint or limb can be moved in the absence of voluntary contraction.

a full squat, spinal side bending while side-lying, or hyper-extension of the wrist when kneeling on all fours. In many of these postures, body weight provides the forces necessary to attain the passive ranges.

Active end-range

The active end-range is predominantly determined by the contraction forces generated by the muscles and the resistance from the antagonistic tissues. As movement approaches the end-range the agonist muscle's contraction force tends to diminish progressively while, conversely, the passive resistance from antagonistic tissues tends to rise (Fig. 2.2).

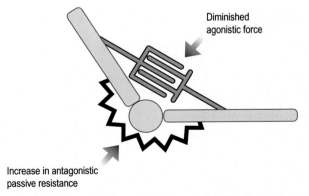

FIGURE 2.2 Active range of movement is limited by a fall in the forces generated by the agonistic muscles owing to excessive filament overlap, and an increase in passive resistance in the antagonistic tissues.

Several factors can influence the active end-range. If you actively extend your index finger the range will be different depending on whether the wrist is held in flexion or extension; so positioning of adjacent joints/limb plays an important part in this range. Also, if you repeat the movement several times, fatigue will set in and you may find that the full range is progressively more difficult to attain. There are many other factors that can affect the active end-range: abnormal shortening of connective tissues, local sensitivity, pain, muscle atrophy, loss of motor control, excessive activity in the antagonistic pair, fear of movement, and many more. So the active end-range is highly variable. But what about the passive end-range? Is it absolute?

Passive end-range

In most joints, the passive ROM is a measure of the individual's tolerance to discomfort or pain and not a true measure of range (Fig. 2.1). If you pull your index finger into extension the end-range will be determined by how much you can tolerate discomfort or pain (see stretch tolerance, Ch. 10). If a goniometer was at hand this position would be measured as the full extension range. However, the extension range would increase further if we were to anaesthetize the area and apply a greater force. So the painful range does not necessarily represent the full biomechanical range. This would apply to joints in which end-ranges are limited by soft-tissue resistance such as the spine, shoulder, hip and ankle, but not where there is bony apposition, such as in elbow extension.

So passive end-range is determined by stretch tolerance, which, by itself, can be highly variable and influenced by numerous factors. For example, sensitivity has natural variations during the day; a stretch performed with discomfort in the morning may be easier in the evening. An individual who stretches regularly will often complain of "good" and "bad" agility days. Sensitivity can change transiently simply as a result of repeating the same movement several times. Stretch the index finger into extension and then repeat it. On the second stretch you will find that it extends further with less discomfort (see creep deformation, Ch. 4). This means that the passive end-range is a vague clinical construct, highly variable and not an absolute measurement as we are often led to believe.[6]

ROM and sensitivity

End-ranges become even more blurred in conditions in which ROM losses are accompanied by pain and sensitization. In these conditions there is reduced tolerance to stretching and the experience of pain and stiffness determines the end-ranges. As a consequence, passive and active ROM losses can be due to elevated stretch sensitivity, but without physical changes in the length or stiffness of the tissues. For example, patients with low back pain often complain of increased spinal and hamstring stiffness in forward bending. However, they have the same flexion ROM as asymptomatic individuals.[7-10] Hence, stretching the back and the legs, a common exercise given to patients with chronic back pain, is unlikely to have any therapeutic value (since nothing is short, it just feels like it).

The variability of tolerance can complicate and add uncertainty to ROM assessment and treatment. We can never be sure how much of the ROM loss is due to "real" biomechanical limitations or is simply because the patient cannot tolerate the discomfort. Furthermore, because the end-range is experiential and not a mechanical phenomenon it provides inaccurate feedback during stretching; it can be difficult to determine how much force to use during stretching. If the area is highly sensitized the patient may terminate the stretching long before it reaches effective levels. Pain and sensitivity can also confuse the treatment progression. Unpredictable adverse reactions and fluctuating sensitivity can overshadow positive biological–adaptive ROM changes. A further discussion of this topic can be found in Chapters 9 and 10.

DEFINING FUNCTIONAL AND DYSFUNCTIONAL ROM

A patient who presented to my clinic complained of several months of moderate shoulder discomfort during the night. On examination, there was total loss of external rotation on the affected side, but all other ROMs were normal. Interestingly, the patient was unaware that she had such profound ROM losses, in particular as she was still able to carry out all her daily activities to the full. She was only concerned about the pain that kept her awake at night.

This case suggests that ROM can be evaluated by using a clinical-anatomical and functional reference points. A clinical-anatomical model often uses the unaffected side or published ROM values as a reference for comparison.[11-16] A functional assessment explores how ROM changes impact the patient's ability to perform a range of daily activities. These two forms of evaluation are not necessarily linked and the functional one is often more important in defining recovery. But what do we mean by functional ROM?

Functional ROM

Functional movement is *the unique movement repertoire of an individual* (Fig. 2.3).[17] This repertoire contains some shared movement patterns associated with daily needs and demands such as feeding, grooming and travelling. Some of the functional repertoire is particular to the individual, containing specialized occupational and recreational activities or sport pursuits.

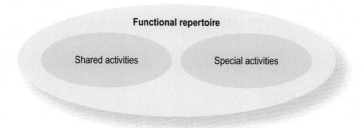

FIGURE 2.3 Functional movements contain the movement repertoire of the individual. This includes universal shared activities and special occupational and recreational activities, which are unique to the individual.

Within functional movement is the person's *functional ROM*. It is the ROM required to perform functional activities effectively, efficiently and comfortably;[18] to have sufficient ROM to reach for a shelf, bend to lift or hip flexibility to walk (shared activities), or the extra flexibility needed for a dancer to perform full splits (special activities).

Most individuals use a relatively small percentage of their full active ROM when performing shared activities (Fig. 2.4).[1-5,19] Hence, these are often performed within a comfort zone, with relative ease and without any stretch discomfort or pain. Infrequently, some shared activities may challenge the margins of this comfort zone, such as the full lumbar flexion required to pick an object off the floor or the full cervical rotation needed for reversing the car.[1,2,19] Special activities, such as yoga or dance, require greater functional

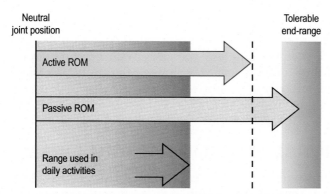

FIGURE 2.4 In many areas of the body daily activities are performed within a small proportion of the active range. Occasionally the full active range is engaged. Passive end-ranges are less often engaged during daily activities. This is why recovery of active range of movement (ROM) should be the focus of rehabilitation.

ROM and are often expected to be performed with some level of discomfort and effort. How far a person chooses to move into ranges that are uncomfortable and even painful depends on their movement goals and pain tolerance. These individuals may consider movement in this extended zone to be normal and even desirable.

Dysfunctional ROM

Often a person will become aware of ROM losses when they are no longer able to perform functional activities to the full. Hence, the use of functionality as a reference point can also help to define dysfunctional ROM: *ROM limitation that impedes the ability to perform functional movement.*

The value an individual gives to any ROM loss is closely related to how adversely it affects their functionality. ROM losses that affect shared activities are obvious, noticeable and likely to be considered dysfunctional by the person concerned. An example would be loss of hip extension affecting walking ability. However, a small loss of full shoulder flexion may go undetected unless the person is attempting to perform a special activity, such as painting a ceiling or doing a handstand. Furthermore, a minor ROM loss for one individual may be experienced as a serious impediment for another. The loss of full shoulder flexion would be more limiting and distressing for a dancer than, say, a footballer. So whether ROM is functional or dysfunctional is determined by the individual's expectations and the requirement of their functional repertoire.

This brings us back to the original question in the introduction; is the lack of flexion ROM in forward bending functional or dysfunctional? That depends on what the person is trying to achieve. There is no ROM "pathology" as long as the stiffer individual is comfortable and able to perform daily activities that require some degree of forward flexion, such as putting on their socks. They are still likely to be within their functional ROM even if they take up a new sport that does not require any special forward bending flexibility, such as running. If they took up yoga their limited flexion ROM would become an impediment, but only in relation to this new activity. Their other shared daily activities would remain unaffected and therefore functional.

FUNCTIONAL AND CLINICAL ROM IDEALS

The use of functionality as a reference point can also help to define treatment success and to some extent determine the treatment ending.

Most patients commence their therapeutic journey in the hope of regaining their health; ideally, as they were before the onset of their condition. Functionality is often their reference point for evaluating improvements and treatment success. This may even be in the absence of full ROM recovery. For example, a patient with frozen shoulder may recover full functionality, but on examination the therapist observes a residual 15–20° loss of flexion. The patient considers the treatment a success but the therapist with the medical knowledge does not. It could be argued that, since this residual loss does not impede functionality, recovering it remains a clinical ideal but an irrelevance to the patient. For example, it was found that after knee replacement the majority of patients obtained a flexion greater than 115° while some obtained flexion greater than 125°.[20] However, there was no difference between the two groups on functionality scores.

So what do we do, terminate the treatment once functionality is attained or continue until ROM is fully recovered? Ultimately, the decision depends on the patient's expectations and how the loss limits their functional repertoire. But it also depends on their knowledge of their condition and their beliefs about flexibility. Many patients (and therapists) believe that residual losses will result in some joint pathology and disability later in life. Because of this fear some will pursue the clinical ROM ideal and choose to continue the treatment. These fears can be alleviated by reassuring the patient that such long-term consequences are unlikely and that, in time, normal daily use will promote recovery. So, often a *well-informed* patient would choose to end the treatment when the ROM has *sufficiently* recovered to perform functional tasks. However, some patients' expectations are set within the clinical ideals. They would like to have full ROM.

All this does not exclude the possibility that in some situations the clinical ROM ideals are essential treatment goals, i.e. full ROM recovery beyond what is needed for full functionality. However, as I write this text I am struggling to recall any clinical example where this was the case.

SUMMARY

- In healthy individuals active ROM is often determined by the inability of an agonist muscle to overcome antagonistic tissue tension. Passive ROM is limited by experience of discomfort and pain (in joints where there is no bony apposition)
- ROM contains active and passive components set within variable and (often) ill-defined end-ranges
- Functional movement is the unique movement repertoire of an individual
- Functional movement contains shared activities, which are universal to all, and special activities, which are specific to each individual
- Functional ROM is defined as the ROM required to perform functional activities effectively, efficiently and comfortably

- Dysfunctional ROM is defined as the ROM limitation that impedes the ability to perform functional movement
- Most daily activities are performed within the active ROM. This suggests that the ROM challenges should also be active and in ranges that support the individual's functional needs
- There are therapists' clinical ROM ideals and patients' functional ROM expectations
- Clinical ROM ideals are based on striving for perfection in physiological ROM and may not reflect the patient's expectations and needs
- Functional ROM expectations are patient-centred movement goals and therefore form the basis for ROM rehabilitation

REFERENCES

1. Bible JE, Biswas D, Miller CP, et al. Normal functional range of motion of the cervical spine during 15 activities of daily living. J Spinal Disord Tech 2010;23(1):15–21.
2. Bible JE, Biswas D, Miller CP, et al. Normal functional range of motion of the lumbar spine during 15 activities of daily living. J Spinal Disord Tech 2010;23(2):106–12.
3. Sardelli M, Tashjian RZ, MacWilliams BA. Functional elbow range of motion for contemporary tasks. J Bone Joint Surg Am 2011;93(5):471–7.
4. Vasen AP, Lacey SH, Keith MW, et al. Functional range of motion of the elbow. J Hand Surg Am 1995;20(2):288–92.
5. Namdari S, Yagnik G, Ebaugh DD, et al. Defining functional shoulder range of motion for activities of daily living. J Shoulder Elbow Surg 2012;21(9):1177–83.
6. Nigg BM, Nigg CR, Reinschmidt C. Reliability and validity of active, passive and dynamic range of motion tests. Sportverletz Sportschaden 1995;9(2):51–7.
7. Esola MA, McClure PW, Fitzgerald GK, et al. Analysis of lumbar spine and hip motion during forward bending in subjects with and without a history of low back pain. Spine 1996;21(1):71–8.
8. Johnson EN, Thomas JS. Effect of hamstring flexibility on hip and lumbar spine joint excursions during forward-reaching tasks in participants with and without low back pain. Arch Phys Med Rehabil 1996;91(7):1140–2.
9. Hultman G, Saraste H, Ohlsen H. Anthropometry, spinal canal width, and flexibility of the spine and hamstring muscles in 45–55-year-old men with and without low back pain. J Spinal Disord 1992;5(3):245–53.
10. Sullivan MS, Shoaf LD, Riddle DL. The relationship of lumbar flexion to disability in patients with low back pain. Phys Ther 2000;80(3):240–50.
11. Macedo LG, Magee DJ. Differences in range of motion between dominant and nondominant sides of upper and lower extremities. J Manipulative Physiol Ther 2008;31(8):577–82.
12. Soucie JM, Wang C, Forsyth A, et al. Range of motion measurements: reference values and a database for comparison studies. Haemophilia 2011;17(3):500–7.
13. Intolo P, Milosavljevic S, Baxter DG, et al. The effect of age on lumbar range of motion: a systematic review. Man Ther 2009;14(6):596–604.
14. Yukawa Y, Kato F, Suda K, et al. Age-related changes in osseous anatomy, alignment, and range of motion of the cervical spine. Part I. Radiographic data from over 1,200 asymptomatic subjects. Eur Spine J 2012;21(8):1492–8.
15. Brown JC, Miller CJ, Schwellnus MP, et al. Range of motion measurements diverge with increasing age for COL5A1 genotypes. Scand J Med Sci Sports 2011;21(6):e266–72.

16. Kumar S, Sharma R, Gulati D, et al. Normal range of motion of hip and ankle in Indian population. Acta Orthop Traumatol Turc 2011;45(6):421–4.
17. Lederman E. Neuromuscular rehabilitation in manual and physical therapy. Edinburgh: Elsevier; 2010.
18. Vasen AP, Lacey SH, Keith MW, et al. Functional range of motion of the elbow. J Hand Surg Am 1995;20(2):288–92.
19. Cobian DG, Sterling AC, Anderson PA, et al. Task-specific frequencies of neck motion measured in healthy young adults over a five-day period. Spine 2009;34(6):E202–7.
20. Meneghini RM, Pierson JL, Bagsby D, et al. Is there a functional benefit to obtaining high flexion after total knee arthroplasty? J Arthroplasty 2007;22(6 Suppl 2):43–6.

CHAPTER 3

Causes of ROM Loss and Therapeutic Potential of Rehabilitation

A patient with a stiff frozen shoulder, an elderly patient with severe cervical spine degeneration and rotation loss, a stroke patient with hand–wrist contractures, a person with Dupuytren's contractures and a patient with post-immobilization range of movement (ROM) limitation: who is likely to benefit from ROM rehabilitation and to what extent?

ROM loss is often the outcome of a condition but rarely its cause. Therapeutic outcome is determined largely by the potential for recovery of the causal condition. It also depends on the capacity of treatment to influence the resolution of the causal condition and its capacity to stimulate the adaptive mechanisms underlying ROM recovery. A patient with central nervous system (CNS) damage (cause) may develop contractures (outcome). Stretching the contracture (outcome) does not normalize the abnormal motor control which maintains the condition (cause). In this case stretching alone without motor rehabilitation is likely to be ineffective. On the other hand, frozen shoulder (cause) is associated with capsular contractures (outcome). Since frozen shoulder is a self-limiting condition it is expected that treating the outcome (shortening) will facilitate ROM recovery.[1]

Hence, identifying the cause and outcome and whether the underlying condition is self-limiting or persistent will have an impact on the treatment priorities, choice of management and the prognosis as well as managing the therapist's and patient's expectations. It is also essential for delimiting the clinical use of ROM rehabilitation.

This chapter will explore the following topics:

- What are the common causes of ROM losses?
- What physiological processes are associated with ROM losses?
- When is ROM loss recoverable?
- When is ROM rehabilitation useful?
- Is stretching always necessary to recover ROM?

25

DEFINING THE BOUNDARY OF ROM REHABILITATION

There are two key factors that determine whether ROM rehabilitation will be therapeutically useful (Fig. 3.1). The first consideration is the prognostic path of the causative condition: whether it is self-limiting, persistent or progressive. Another consideration is the condition's potential for repair and adaptation as well as symptomatic relief: the three processes that underlie ROM recovery (Ch. 1). When these processes are preserved, ROM rehabilitation is likely to be more successful than in those conditions in which they are disrupted by the disease process.

Self-limiting conditions

Acute tissue damage is one of the most common self-limiting causes of ROM loss. In many forms of injury, tissue damage is not associated with *tissue short-ening or stiffening*. The limitation in movement is often due to internal swelling within the affected tissues combined with a complex protective strategy that includes pain, increased sensitivity and motor reorganization of movement.[2,3] Such acute ROM loss can be seen in delayed onset muscle soreness (DOMS)

Potential for adaptation/repair

		Preserved	Lost
Condition	Self-limiting	Post-immobilization Post-surgery Frozen shoulder Tendinopathies?	
	Persistent	Postural Post-stroke Scoliosis	Burns Autoimmune
	Progressive	CNS disease	Dupuytren's contractures Autoimmune

FIGURE 3.1 Classification of the prognosis path of the condition in relation to potential for adaptation and repair. CNS, central nervous system.

after exercise, a mild form of muscle damage.[4] Stiffness and ROM losses develop very rapidly within days after exercising, last for a few days and recover fully in line with muscle repair. The patient's subjective experience of stiffness/ROM loss is due to swelling and sensitivity and a loss in force production. Since in acute injuries there is no "true" shortening of tissues the therapeutic aim is to support the tissue repair processes. This can be facilitated by passive or active movement *within pain-free ranges* (see Ch. 9).[5] Although stretching is widely used by therapists and athletes to treat ROM losses following acute injuries or DOMS, it is unnecessary and may even be detrimental.[6,7]

Inactivity or restricted movement range is another common cause of ROM losses. This outcome is often seen after prolonged disabling injuries, post-surgery and following immobilization. In this spectrum of conditions the ROM losses are an adaptive response, secondary to the underlying condition. The shortened, inextensible tissues often preserve their capacity for adaptation and therefore have a good potential to recover to a pre-injury state, depending on various factors such as the magnitude of damage (Ch. 4). In this group of conditions, ROM challenges are likely to be useful.

Between the self-limiting and persistent conditions are several conditions in which pain and sensitization give rise to the experience of stiffness and ROM loss; yet, there is no true shortening of the affected area (Ch. 9).[8,9] This phenomenon is observed in many long-term conditions such as chronic back and neck pain,[10,11] trapezius myalgia[12,13] and many of the tendinopathies such as tennis elbow, plantar fasciitis and Achilles tendinosis.[14–18] In this spectrum of conditions, pain alleviation and desensitization may also be associated with adaptation within the nociceptive system. Stretching may have little or no effect on these processes and other forms of management should be considered, such as the use of relaxation or working with fear-related cognitions. This group of conditions and their management are discussed in more detail in Chapters 9 and 11.

Persistent conditions

Within the persistent group are ROM changes which are associated with behavioural, non-pathological conditions. There is a widely held belief that prolonged restrictive postural sets/behavioural patterns will result in tissue shortening. For example, some people believe that prolonged sitting with hunched shoulders will result in protracted scapula and shortened pectoral muscles. However, there is very little support for this from the sciences. It seems that even small breaks from the causal activity will offset or "normalize" these imbalances (Ch. 7).[19] There are occasional exceptions, such as the association between regular wearing of high-heel shoes with shortening of the calf muscle and modest ROM restriction in the ankle.[20]

In this group of conditions the adaptive capacity is fully preserved. Hence, if such shortening is evident it can be easily resolved by modifying the causal activity, for example by wearing flat shoes or changing sitting posture. Traditional stretching methods are likely to be ineffective and short-lasting unless there is a concomitant change in movement behaviour. So some ROM recovery can just be about a change in behaviour.

Certain occupational and sports activities may also result in low-level ROM changes in specific joints and movement planes.[21-24] These changes often represent positive, sport-specific ROM adaptations that are beneficial for optimum performance. For example, runners tend to have stiffer lower limbs, which is believed to be a positive adaptation related to movement economy.[25] Similarly, baseball players may develop minor changes in scapular position and motion.[26] In these forms of adaptation, tissue changes are often minor and unlikely to have a negative impact on daily activities. Importantly, there is no pathology here and it might be imprudent to interfere with such beneficial sport-specific adaptation. There is no clinical or physiological value in stretching and it may even reduce sports performance.[27-32]

Scoliosis also falls within the persistent category. Correction of this benign postural state has been the target of many failed manual and physical stretching approaches (it might be the time to give up).[33] Post-surgical complications, severe adhesions and surgical shortening of tissue can result in permanent, non-progressive ROM losses. In such non-progressive conditions some ROM recovery may be possible, particularly if it is adaptive and secondary to the condition (such as from disuse). However, this recovery, too, depends on the extent of damage/repair and the tissues' capacity for adaptation.

Non-progressive CNS damage, such as stroke and head trauma, can result in persistent dysfunctional movement control that may lead to joint contractures.[34-40] It has been estimated that up to 6 hours of daily stretching is required to compete with the chronic neuromuscular drive that maintains the shortening (see competition in adaptation, Ch. 7).[35] In these conditions the therapeutic focus should be on recovering motor control (cause). ROM rehabilitation is unlikely to be effective without such improvement.[34] This can be exemplified in a case of a stroke patient who presented with severe hand and wrist contractures. Initially, his carer could only open the clenched fist by using full force and throwing her body weight behind it. This strategy was used for 5 years without any obvious improvement. Over a period of a few months he was taught to relax the arm and was eventually able to open the clenched hand fully without any stretching (but with some assistance). Interestingly, once this control was achieved he was able to permanently maintain the relaxed hand position throughout the day and night. So some ROM rehabilitation is about motor control rather than stretching.

Progressive conditions

The most prevalent progressive ROM loss is seen in ageing.[41-43] ROM tends to decline irregularly, affecting particular movement planes and specific joints.[43-45] For example, in the lumbar spine flexion and extension ROMs tend to decline but not rotation ROM.[43,44] Some range loss may be partly adaptive owing to disuse and loss of force production necessary to achieve full active end-ranges. Some of these losses can be recovered by stretching as well as resistance training.[46-49] However, these force–flexibility gains are notoriously difficult to adhere to and rapidly vanish when the training is terminated (competition in adaptation),[48] in particular for an elderly individual who is adopting a progressively sedentary lifestyle and may have other health problems.

There are numerous persistent and progressive conditions that lead to ROM losses. They include degenerative musculoskeletal disease (e.g. osteoarthritis), progressive CNS pathologies (e.g. muscular dystrophies, Parkinson's disease),[50] Dupuytren's contractures and autoimmune conditions, such as rheumatoid arthritis and scleroderma.[51] In this group of conditions rehabilitation may improve ROM marginally and temporarily,[51] but is unlikely to prevent ROM losses in the long term. The therapist should consider a multidisciplinary approach in which ROM rehabilitation is combined with other forms of therapy to help resolve the underlying condition.

In summary, ROM rehabilitation is likely to be effective in self-limiting conditions in which the affected tissues have maintained their adaptive or reparative capacity (Fig. 3.2). In these situations the aim is to help the patient recover

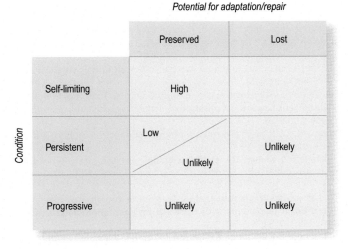

FIGURE 3.2 Potential for range of movement recovery.

functionality within the shortest time possible. This therapeutic potential diminishes in persistent and progressive conditions, particularly when the recovery mechanisms have been affected by disease processes.

SUMMARY

- ROM loss is often the outcome/symptom of a condition
- The conditions that cause ROM loss can be classified as self-limiting, persistent or progressive
- ROM recovery is dependent on repair and adaptation (and symptomatic relief)
- ROM rehabilitation is likely to be more effective in conditions where the adaptive and reparative capacity of the affected tissues is saved
- ROM rehabilitation will have a diminishing effect in persistent and progressive conditions, in particular if the adaptive or reparative capacity of the affected tissue is reduced

REFERENCES

1. Hand C, Clipsham K, Rees JL, et al. Long-term outcome of frozen shoulder. J Shoulder Elbow Surg 2008;17(2):231–6.
2. Mayer J, Graves JE, Clark BC, et al. The use of magnetic resonance imaging to evaluate lumbar muscle activity during trunk extension exercise at varying intensities. Spine 2005; 30(22):2556–63.
3. Lederman E. Neuromuscular rehabilitation in manual and physical therapies. Edinburgh: Elsevier; 2010.
4. Reinold MM, Wilk KE, Macrina LC, et al. Changes in shoulder and elbow passive range of motion after pitching in professional baseball players. Am J Sports Med 2008;36(3):523–7.
5. Lederman E. The science and practice of manual therapy. Edinburgh: Elsevier; 2005.
6. Herbert RD, de Noronha M, Kamper SJ. Stretching to prevent or reduce muscle soreness after exercise. Cochrane Database Syst Rev 2011;7:CD004577.
7. Andersen JC. Stretching before and after exercise: effect on muscle soreness and injury risk. J Athl Train 2005;40(3):218–20.
8. Schaible HG, Richter F, Ebersberger A, et al. Joint pain. Exp Brain Res 2009;196(1):153–62.
9. Woolf CJ. Central sensitization: implications for the diagnosis and treatment of pain. Pain 2011;152(Suppl. 3):S2–15.
10. Hoy DG, Protani M, De R, et al. The epidemiology of neck pain. Best Pract Res Clin Rheumatol 2010;24(6):783–92.
11. Hush JM, Michaleff Z, Maher CG, et al. Individual, physical and psychological risk factors for neck pain in Australian office workers: a 1-year longitudinal study. Eur Spine J 2009;18(10): 1532–40.
12. Rosendale L, Larsson B, Kristiansen J, et al. Increase in muscle nociceptive substances and anaerobic metabolism in patients with trapezius myalgia: microdialysis in rest and during exercise. Pain 2004;112(3):324–34.
13. Sjøgaard G, Rosendal L, Kristiansen J, et al. Muscle oxygenation and glycolysis in females with trapezius myalgia during stress and repetitive work using microdialysis and NIRS. Eur J Appl Physiol 2010;108(4):657–69.

14. Zeisig E, Ohberg L, Alfredson H. Extensor origin vascularity related to pain in patients with tennis elbow. Knee Surg Sports Traumatol Arthrosc 2006;14(7):659–63.

15. Yu JS, Popp JE, Kaeding CC, et al. Correlation of MR imaging and pathologic findings in athletes undergoing surgery for chronic patellar tendinitis. Am J Roentgenol 1995;165(1):115–18.

16. Alfredson H. Chronic tendon pain – implications for treatment: an update. Curr Drug Targets 2004;5(5):407–10.

17. Rolf CG, Fu BSC, Pau A, et al. Increased cell proliferation and associated expression of PDGFRβ causing hypercellularity in patellar tendinosis. Rheumatology 2001;40:256–61.

18. Walz DM, Newman JS, Konin GP, et al. Epicondylitis: pathogenesis, imaging, and treatment. Radiographics 2010;30(1):167–84.

19. Hrysomallis C, Goodman C. A review of resistance exercise and posture realignment. J Strength Cond Res 2001;15(3):385–90.

20. Csapo R, Maganaris CN, Seynnes OR, et al. On muscle, tendon and high heels. J Exp Biol 2010;213(Pt 15):2582–8.

21. Travers PR, Evans PG. Annotation limitation of mobility in major joints of 231 sportsmen. Br J Sports Med 1976;10(1):35–6.

22. Wright RW, Steger-May K, Wasserlauf BL, et al. Elbow range of motion in professional baseball pitchers. Am J Sports Med 2006;34(2):190–3.

23. Ellenbecker TS, Roetert EP, Bailie DS, et al. Glenohumeral joint total rotation range of motion in elite tennis players and baseball pitchers. Med Sci Sports Exerc 2002;34(12):2052–6.

24. Bigliani LU, Codd TP, Connor PM, et al. Shoulder motion and laxity in the professional baseball player. Am J Sports Med 1997;25(5):609–13.

25. Gleim GW, McHugh MP. Flexibility and its effects on sports injury and performance. Sports Med 1997;24(5):289–99.

26. Thomas SJ, Swanik KA, Swanik CB, et al. Internal rotation and scapular position differences: a comparison of collegiate and high school baseball players. J Athl Train 2010;45(1):44–50.

27. Shrier I. Does stretching improve performance? A systematic and critical review of the literature. Clin J Sport Med 2004;14(5):267–73.

28. Witvrouw E, Mahieu N, Danneels L, et al. Stretching and injury prevention: an obscure relationship. Sports Med 2004;34(7):443–9.

29. Gremion G. Is stretching for sports performance still useful? A review of the literature. Rev Med Suisse 2005;1(28):1830–4.

30. Behm DG, Button DC, Butt JC. Factors affecting force loss with prolonged stretching. Appl Physiol 2001;26(3):261–72.

31. Young WB, Behm DG. Should static stretching be used during a warm-up for strength and power activities? Strength Cond J 2002;24:33–7.

32. Rubini EC, Costa AL, Gomes PS. The effects of stretching on strength performance. Sports Med 2007;37:213–24.

33. Lederman E. The fall of the postural–structural–biomechanical model in manual and physical therapies: exemplified by lower back pain. J Bodyw Mov Ther 2011;15(2):131–8.

34. Hufschmidt A, Mauritz KH. Chronic transformation of muscle in spasticity: a peripheral contribution to increased tone. J Neurol Neurosurg Psychiatry 1985;48(7):676–85.

35. Tardieu C, Lespargot A, Tabary C, et al. For how long must the soleus muscle be stretched each day to prevent contracture? Dev Med Child Neurol 1988;30:3–10.

36. Katz RT, Rymer WZ. Spastic hypertonia: mechanisms and measurement. Arch Phys Med Rehabil 1989;70(2):144–55.

37. Hidler JM, Carroll M, Federovich EH. Strength and coordination in the paretic leg of individuals following acute stroke. IEEE Trans Neural Syst Rehabil Eng 2007;15(4):526–34.

38. Levin MF, Selles RW, Verheul MH, et al. Deficits in the coordination of agonist and antagonist muscles in stroke patients: implications for normal motor control. Brain Res 2000;853(2):352–69.

39. O'Dwyer NJ, Ada L, Neilson PD. Spasticity and muscle contracture following stroke. Brain 1996;119(Pt 5):1737–49.
40. Ada L, Canning CG, Low SL. Stroke patients have selective muscle weakness in shortened range. Brain 2003;126(Pt 3):724–31.
41. Steultjens MPM, Dekker J, van Baar ME. Range of joint motion and disability in patients with osteoarthritis of the knee or hip. Rheumatology 2000;39(9):955–61.
42. Simpson AK, Biswas D, Emerson JW, et al. Quantifying the effects of age, gender, degeneration, and adjacent level degeneration on cervical spine range of motion using multivariate analyses. Spine 2008;33(2):183–6.
43. Bible JE, Simpson AK, Emerson JW, et al. Quantifying the effects of degeneration and other patient factors on lumbar segmental range of motion using multivariate analysis. Spine 2008;33(16):1793–9.
44. Intolo P, Milosavljevic S, Baxter DG, et al. The effect of age on lumbar range of motion: a systematic review. Man Ther 2009;14(6):596–604.
45. Tommasi DG, Foppiani AC, Galante D, et al. Active head and cervical range of motion: effect of age in healthy females. Spine 2009;34(18):1910–16.
46. Barbosa AR, Santarém JM, Filho WJ, et al. Effects of resistance training on the sit-and-reach test in elderly women. J Strength Cond Res 2002;16(1):14–18.
47. Monteiro WD, Simão R, Polito MD, et al. Influence of strength training on adult women's flexibility. J Strength Cond Res 2008;22(3):672–7.
48. Fatouros IG, Kambas A, Katrabasas I, et al. Resistance training and detraining effects on flexibility performance in the elderly are intensity-dependent. J Strength Cond Res 2006;20(3):634–42.
49. Simão R, Lemos A, Salles B, et al. The influence of strength, flexibility, and simultaneous training on flexibility and strength gains. J Strength Cond Res 2011;25(5):1333–8.
50. Hu MT, Bland J, Clough C, et al. Limb contractures in levodopa-responsive parkinsonism: a clinical and investigational study of seven new cases. J Neurol 1999;246(8):671–6.
51. Poole JL. Musculoskeletal rehabilitation in the person with scleroderma. Curr Opin Rheumatol 2010;22(2):205–12.

Adaptation in ROM Loss and Recovery

The capacity of the musculoskeletal system to undergo range of movement (ROM) adaptation can be seen in a number of human experiences, from the dramatic elongation of the anterior abdominal wall in pregnancy and the gains of flexibility in yoga and dance to ROM losses during immobilization and ROM recovery during rehabilitation. These adaptive processes are whole-person changes that can be observed in the tissue, neurological and psychological dimensions (Fig. 4.1).

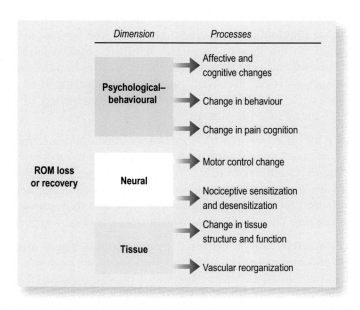

FIGURE 4.1 Adaptation in range of movement (ROM) loss and recovery is multidimensional. Adaptation in the neurological and psychological dimensions is discussed in Chapters 8, 9 and 11.

This chapter will explore the following topics:

- What is the physiology of adaptation?
- What happens to tissues during ROM loss?
- How do tissues adapt in ROM recovery?
- What drives adaptation?

The focus in this chapter will be primarily on adaptation in the tissue dimension, using immobilization and post-injury and post-surgery conditions as a model to explore ROM loss and recovery.

THE WONDERS OF MECHANOTRANSDUCTION

Underlying the body's adaptive capacity is a physiological mechanism called *mechanotransduction*. It is a mechanism whereby the body converts mechanical signals into biological processes.[1-18] A notable example of mechanotransduction is the musculoskeletal adaptation seen in response to sports training. Mechanotransduction is also the process underlying the tissue changes observed during ROM loss and recovery.

Within the musculoskeletal system the masters of mechanotransduction are the myocytes and fibroblasts (often called mechanocytes). They produce the various biological materials that compose the tissues in which they are found.[19,20] These physiological functions are modulated by the physical stress that is imposed on the tissues. Recurrent, habitual physical loading results in higher synthesis and turnover of these biological materials and lowered turnover during inactivity.[21] Generally, mechanotransduction is more readily stimulated when connective tissue and muscle are preloaded in tension – the essence of many ROM challenges.[22,23]

More recently the interface at which mechanotransduction occurs has been identified as the attachment points between the fibroblasts' and myocytes' cell surfaces to the extra-cellular matrix.[20,24,25] At these sites there are specialized proteins that act as mechanical sensors. When a stretch is applied, the deformation of the tissue activates membrane channels that convert the mechanical signals into chemical signals within the cells (Fig. 4.2).[20,25]

Mechanotransduction can be activated by mechanical signal alone in the absence of blood or nerve supply. This phenomenon can be demonstrated in denervated muscle and laboratory samples of muscle or isolated fibroblast/connective tissue.[26,27] This highlights the significance of physical stress in shaping adaptation; a salient message for ROM rehabilitation.

The mechanical signals that stimulate mechanotransduction activate a cascade of cellular events that continue long after the cessation of stimulation.

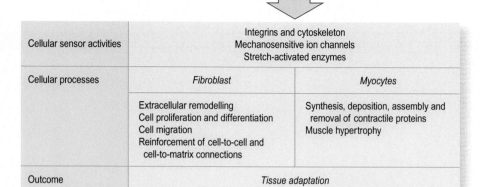

FIGURE 4.2 Processes associated with mechanotransduction.

This phenomenon can be observed following resistance training.[18] Muscle hypertrophy (biological dimension) does not occur during the training session (biomechanical dimension), but later, long after the cessation of exercise and including times when the person is resting. For example, a peak release of mechanogrowth factor can be observed in the human forearm muscles 2 hours after eccentric exercise.[15] A similar phenomenon can be observed in connective tissue after the cessation of stretching or exercise. Fibroblast activity and reorientation of collagen fibres can be observed after several hours; it peaks at 24 hours and can remain elevated for up to 3 days.[21,28]

DYSFUNCTIONAL ADAPTATION AND ROM LOSSES

ROM loss is a form of dysfunctional adaptive reorganization that takes place when loading forces change or drop below a functional threshold (Fig. 4.3). The deleterious influences of underloading/immobilization are pervasive, affecting all musculoskeletal tissues, including the muscle–tendon unit, fascia, ligaments, joint capsule and intracapsular structures such as articular surfaces and synovium (Fig. 4.4).[29–34]

Connective tissue and intracapsular structures

There are several mechanisms associated with the loss of ROM during immobilization. The loss of extensibility is partly due to collagen fibres adhering to each other by chemical bonds called *cross-linking*.[35] Under normal circumstances, the collagen fibres are intermingled with a gel, containing

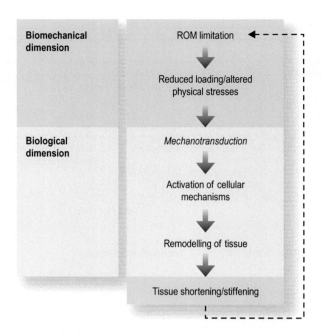

FIGURE 4.3 The transition from biomechanical to biological processes as a model for dysfunctional range of movement (ROM) adaptation.

glycosaminoglycans, that has a high water content.[36] This gel provides volume to the collagen matrix, helping to keep the collagen fibres apart, similar to dipping a cotton-bud in water – it tends to swell as the fibres separate. The gel also acts as a lubricant that allows the fibres to glide over each other. During immobilization the gel content tends to decline, resulting in approximation of the fibres and loss of lubrication.[37] As a consequence, the fibres tend to "stick" to each other, and, like glue, will "set" and become progressively strong over several days.[38] This process is more marked during the first 2 weeks after an injury or immobilization, when there is a high turnover of collagen in the tissues.

A similar process underlies adhesion formation. Here, the abnormal deposition of collagen and cross-linking is between gliding surfaces, such as tendons within their sheaths or synovial villi. In animal studies, adhesion of the synovial villi was found to be a major cause of ROM loss during immobilization (Fig. 4.4).[39–43] Longer durations of immobilization result in stronger and more numerous cross-links. The consequence is formation of adhesions that

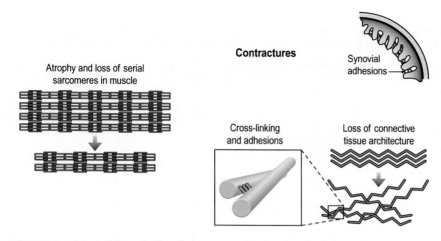

Atrophy and loss of serial
sarcomeres in muscle

Contractures

Synovial
adhesions

Cross-linking
and adhesions

Loss of connective
tissue architecture

FIGURE 4.4 Some of the adaptive changes associated with immobilization and
contracture.

have greater tensile strength than the tissues to which they are attached. When
this occurs, vigorous stretching may fail to break up the adhesions but may
damage the tissues to which they are attached.

In addition to cross-linking and adhesion tissue extensibility may be reduced
by shortening and reorientation of the collagen fibres (Fig. 4.5).[44,45] Normally,
collagen fibres have a crimp-like structure organized along the lines of tension
in the tissue. During tension loading, some elongation occurs by flattening of
this crimp structure. In immobilization, this crimp architecture is lost. The
normal longitudinal arrangement of the fibres becomes disorganized, forming
a random criss-cross pattern. The outcome is stiffening and weakening of the
tissue (Fig. 4.5).

Not all tissues respond equally to immobilization. Ligaments demonstrate
reduced cross-section, weakening and an increase in compliance (less stiff),
whereas tendons increase in stiffness.[38,46–50] In animals, 8 weeks of immobilization resulted in a 40% decrease in tensile strength and a 55% increase in
ligament compliance.[51] However, this may vary between conditions; for
example, in osteoarthritis of the knee there is an increase in stiffness of the
medial, lateral and collateral ligaments.[52,53]

Clinically, it is difficult to assess tissue strength. There is always an uncertainty
as to how much force we should use during stretching. This uncertainty can

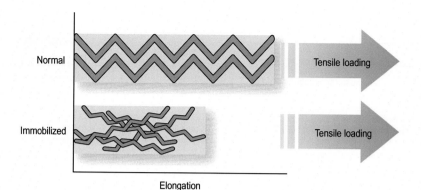

FIGURE 4.5 Loss of connective tissue extensibility can be due to reorientation, loss of crimp structure and shorter fibres.

be overcome by introducing tissue loading in a graded manner over several sessions (see graded challenge, Ch. 6).

Muscle changes

Muscle–tendon adaptation is largely related to the efficiency and effectiveness of force production. Optimal force production is observed when the muscle length corresponds to the resting position of the muscle or neutral position of the joint. Force production is diminished if the muscle has to contract while overstretched or in a shortened position (plotted as the *active force–angle curve*; Fig. 4.6). This change in force (and velocity) generation is related to the overlap of the myofilaments. In the neutral position the cross-bridges are optimally overlapped for force generation, whereas they are excessively overlapped in the shortened position and insufficiently overlapped in the lengthened position.

During immobilization, the neutral position of the joint is displaced and, as a consequence, the muscle has to adapt around this new position.[54] However, the sarcomeres have only a limited capacity to change their length. This is overcome by the muscle's capacity to add or remove sarcomeres to preserve the optimal overlap (Fig. 4.7). This is akin to making a chain longer or shorter by adding or removing links rather than changing the size of the individual links. In a similar manner, sarcomeres are removed when the muscle is immobilized or forced to function in a shortened position, and added in the lengthened positions.[54-64] The loss of sarcomeres in series can be as high as 40% in the shortened muscle, and there may be a 20% gain in the lengthened muscle.[56] This adaptive process was shown to start within hours of immobilization or when the muscle is stimulated to contract in a shortened position/

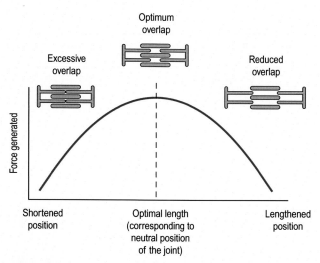

FIGURE 4.6 The active force–angle curve. Force generation is optimal close to neutral joint angles and tends to diminish in the shortened or lengthened positions.

range.[57] The deposition of new sarcomeres can be observed within 4 days of stimulating the muscle.[65]

During the first 2 weeks of immobilization muscle shortening/stiffening plays a larger role in loss of ROM than other joint structures. In animal studies, 2 weeks of joint immobilization resulted in a 20° loss as a result of muscle adaptation compared with a 6.5° loss attributed to joint structures. After that adjustment period, the muscle seems to complete the process of adaptation and "settle" around the angle of immobilization. At that stage it contributes marginally to the contracture. For example, at 32 weeks only a 1.0° loss is attributed to muscle tissue versus a 51.5° loss attributed to connective tissue structures.[39–41]

The reorganization of the muscle length around the position of immobilization is also associated with loss of parallel sarcomeres. The outcome is muscle atrophy and force loss, the essential components of the active ROM. This highlights the importance of introducing active challenges early in the ROM rehabilitation programme.

Connective tissue change in muscle

Normal mechanical links between the muscle cells and their final insertions are essential for optimal transmission of contraction forces.[16,66] This link originates from the attachment of the myofilaments to the connective tissue in the

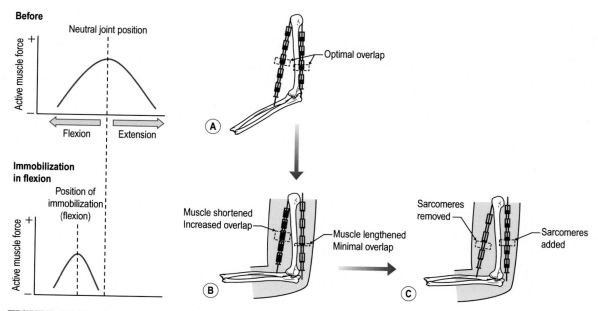

FIGURE 4.7 Muscle contraction is optimized during immobilization or change in use by adding or removing sarcomeres in series. A. Normal. B. Immediately following immobilization there is excessive overlap in the lengthened muscle. C. After a few weeks sarcomeres are removed in the shortened and added in the lengthened muscle.

extra-cellular matrix, to the perimysium and subsequently to the tendon, aponeuroses and bone. Transmission of the contraction force can be impeded by damage or dysfunctional adaptive changes in any part of this connective tissue link (Fig. 4.8).[16,66,67]

Changes in the muscle's connective tissue can be observed during immobilization or partial mobility.[16,66-68] Within the first 2 days after immobilization the ratio of collagen in muscle increases as a result of a rapid loss of muscle fibre (in the shortened but not in the lengthened muscle).[66] Within 4 weeks of immobilization the muscle's fascia can shorten by as much as 25%.[59,60] Interestingly, in this particular study changes in the fascia were also observed in the non-immobilized, control side (15% decrease in the connective tissue length and reorientation of the fibres). This adaptation was associated with the abnormal movement patterns imposed on the animal by the one-sided immobilization. Furthermore, in immobilized muscle, collagen fibres were found to be arranged at a more acute angle to the axis of the muscle fibres than in controls.[66]

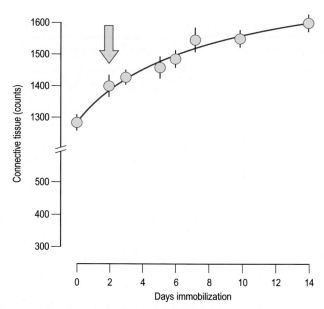

FIGURE 4.8 Connective tissue content of immobilized muscle (endomysium and perimysium). Arrow. Threshold at which there is a significant difference between the experimental and control measurements. *Reprinted from Williams PE, Goldspink G. Connective tissue changes in immobilised muscle. J Anat 1984;138(2):343–50 with permission from John Wiley & Sons.*

ADAPTATION IN ROM RECOVERY

The adaptive recovery of ROM is the story of ROM loss but in reverse (Fig. 4.9).

Recovery in connective tissue

There are two potential mechanisms that could account for ROM recovery: normalization of the tissue's stiffness/compliance or gradual adaptive elongation of the fibres.

During remobilization there are several factors which account for recovery the tissues' extensibility: normalization of the gel content,[37] reduction of abnormal collagen cross-bridges, recovery of the crimp structure, normalizing of fibre reorientation,[28,35,69] and reduced intra-articular adhesions.[70] In ligaments, reorganization of collagen fibres can take place in as little as 6 weeks of remobilization.

How length changes occur in connective tissue is not entirely clear. One potential mechanism is by assembly of collagen fibres in series, similar to the

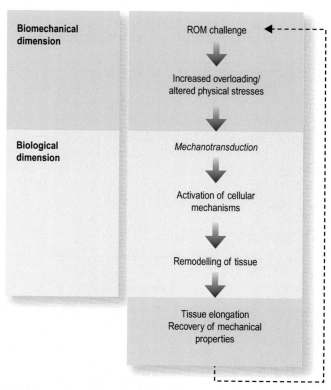

FIGURE 4.9 Adaptive range of movement (ROM) recovery. The transition from biomechanical to biological dimension as a model for tissue-related ROM recovery.

deposition and removal of sarcomeres in muscle. The fibroblasts lead a double life: they construct the tissue's matrix but at the same time produce the enzymes that degrade it. This turnover of collagen is elevated during tensional loading and may account for a length adaptation. A similar length remodelling process is seen in connective tissue during the repair process.[71-76]

Remobilization has the added benefit of improving the tissue's tensile strength by recovering its unique architecture and also by compacting collagen fibrils into thicker and denser bundles.[34,35,77-82] In laboratory samples, stretched collagen was shown to be 10 times stronger, eight-fold denser, and eight times thinner than non-stretched samples.[83]

Generally, connective tissues tend to adapt over long time periods. After immobilization it can take connective tissues several months or longer to regain their mechanical properties.[37,84]

Adaptive recovery in muscle

At a muscular level, ROM rehabilitation is all about shifting the angles of use from the immobilized to the functional ranges. This drives a muscle re-adaptation around newly recovered angles. This functional equilibrium is achieved by normalizing the number of sarcomeres and by muscle hypertrophy (Fig. 4.10). Such changes can be observed in muscle within days of remobilization and within a week there are demonstrable increases in the muscle's length and girth.[23]

The adaptation around the recovered ranges is more likely to occur during active than passive movement.[85] This was demonstrated in a study where subjects were either passively stretched or instructed to perform resistance exercise at the end-range.[86] A shift in the active force–angle curve towards the exercised position was only evident in the active group. This principle can be applied during ROM rehabilitation. Imagine a clinical scenario in which a patient has loss of external rotation in the shoulder. With assistance there is a 10° increase in external rotation. At this newly recovered angle the patient is then instructed to perform a variety of movements. These movements should resemble normal functional activities (Ch. 5). For example, "wash the wall" movement patterns can be used to challenge external rotation. Similarly, adaptation around internal rotation can be driven by "wash the back" movement patterns (see Ch. 12 and video demonstration).

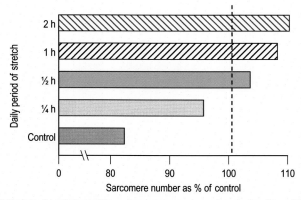

FIGURE 4.10 Removal and deposition of sarcomeres in series during immobilization in the shortened position and daily remobilization in the lengthened position. Control animals were immobilized for 2 weeks. Experimental animals were also immobilized for 2 weeks but remobilized for daily periods of ¼, ½, 1 and 2 hours. Periods of stretching lasting half an hour or more were found to maintain normal dorsiflexion of the ankle as well as to prevent sarcomere loss. *Reproduced from Williams PE. Use of intermittent stretch in the prevention of serial sarcomere loss in immobilised muscle. Ann Rheum Dis 1990;49:316–17 with permission from BMJ Publishing Group Ltd.*

Should these challenges be dynamic or static? This probably depends on the activity that we aim to recover (see specificity of training, Ch. 5). However, there are some indications from laboratory studies that synthesis and deposition of myofilaments in muscle are enhanced by cyclical rather than static loading and more by active than by passive movements.[15,87–90] In animal studies, the synthesis of contractile proteins is dramatically increased when a muscle is stretched and electrically stimulated to contract rhythmically.[15,87–89,91,92] This stimulation is similar to muscle activation during rhythmic daily activities; in particular, when performed at the end-ranges.

Muscle connective tissue

The mechanical properties and content of connective tissue tend to normalize during remobilization.[16,59,60,67] In animal studies, passive stretch of only 15 minutes every other day maintained a normal ratio of muscle to connective tissue as well as prevented the development of connective tissue contractures at the joint (Fig. 4.11).[16]

Here, too, there seems to be an advantage in cyclical, rather than static, loading. In muscle tissue cultures, connective tissue protein synthesis increases by 22% during static and by 38% during cyclical stretching.[90]

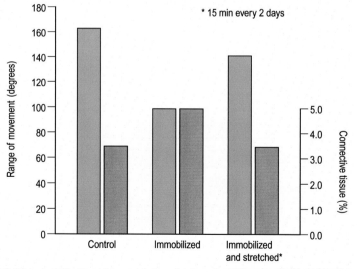

FIGURE 4.11 Immobilization of a muscle in a shortened position results in a reduction of serial sarcomeres and the proportional increase in intramuscular connective tissue. Measurements of ankle ROM show that these changes resulted in a substantial loss of joint flexibility. Fifteen minutes of intermittent passive stretch, every other day was shown to prevent the accumulation of connective tissue in the muscle as well as preventing some of the adaptive connective tissue changes around the joint. *Reproduced from Williams PE. Effect of intermittent stretch on immobilised muscle. Ann Rheum Dis 1988;47:1014–16 with permission from BMJ Publishing Group Ltd.*

ADAPTATION IN OTHER TISSUES/ SYSTEMS/DIMENSIONS

The effects of physical activity and stretching are whole body/person adaptation that can be seen in dimensions and tissues other than connective and muscle tissue.

- **Vascular adaptation** – The epithelial and smooth muscle cells that form the blood and lymph vessels also have mechanotransduction capacity.[93–95] Vascular and lymphatic system reorganization is also observed under tensional forces. In laboratory studies, externally applied stretching was shown to regulate the sprouting of new blood vessels, their length and their alignment in the tissue. In tendon repair studies, movement directs the revascularization and reorientation of the blood vessels in parallel to the tendon; an orientation which is well adapted to withstand the longitudinal forces and gliding of the tendon within its sheath. Conversely, immobilization produces a random misaligned vascular pattern that tends to fail when movement is reintroduced.[35,96]

- **Motor control adaptation** – The loss and recovery of the active ROM is closely related to the adaptive capacity of the motor system.[97–99] These adaptive control changes are extensive and can be observed throughout the central nervous system. This multilevel adaptation has been demonstrated during immobilization. Within the spinal cord there were changes in the firing patterns of the motoneurons as well as in the cortical and cerebellar representations of the immobilized limb.[100–103] Such adaptive motor changes are rapid, and are observed within the first 3 weeks, but probably begin within hours or days of immobilization and active remobilization.[104]

  Motor control changes are expected to normalize rapidly if there are no central nervous system pathologies. In immobilization, the tissues in the periphery may be damaged, but, centrally, the system is fully intact, healthy and therefore has the full capacity to adapt.[99] It is expected that motor control should normalize once activity is resumed.

  Motor control considerations during ROM rehabilitation are further discussed in Chapter 8. (For a full discussion of sensory–motor adaptation, see Lederman.[99])

- **Nociceptive and sensitization adaptation** – Range sensitivity and desensitization are also associated with adaptation within the nociceptive system and psychological dimension. For a full discussion, see Chapters 9 and 11.

- **Psychological/cognitive "adaptation"** – Adaptation in the form of learned association and changes in behaviour is also observed in the psychological dimension. For a full discussion, see Chapter 11.

WHAT (REALLY) DRIVES ADAPTATION IN RECOVERY

The fibroblasts' and myocytes' capacity to convert physical signals into biological processes suggests that physical loading drives adaptation. However, this can be a limited view. "Someone" has to carry out the physical loading, which brings us to behaviour. It is the actions of the individual, their movement patterns, that provide the necessary stresses required for adaptation, i.e. behaviour drives adaptation. But this still remains an incomplete view. We have to consider that behaviour is the product of the individual's mind, their emotions, moods, needs and drives. Whether they are anxious, depressed or motivated will influence their recovery behaviour. For example, a person with movement-related fears may fail to maintain the behaviour that drives this adaptation. Imagine what would happen to the adaptive process if the patient is elderly, has had a mild stroke, lives alone in a small flat, needs walking rehabilitation but is fearful to walk outside? Adaptation can be viewed as a cascade originating at the interface between the individual and their physical, social and cultural environment, their psychological state, expressed physically as behaviour and culminating with tissue loading and activation of mechanotransduction (Fig. 4.12).

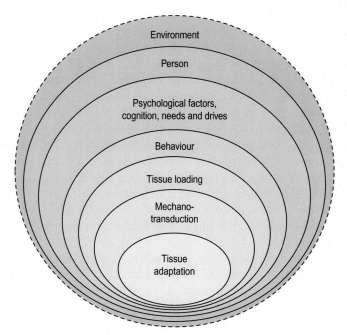

FIGURE 4.12 Adaptation occurs within the context of what the person does within their environment.

This cascade of influences defines the clinical management of ROM recovery. It is about co-creating with the patient environments in which their recovery can be enhanced. It is a multidimensional environment that encompasses lifestyle, social, psychological, cognitive and behavioural factors (Ch. 11). The important message here is that the locus of recovery is intrinsic to the individual and is subject to environmental circumstances. Hence, *the success of ROM rehabilitation is not inherent in any single stretching approach but in the overall management.*

SUMMARY

- ROM loss and recovery is represented by several interlinked processes that occur in the tissue, neurological and psychological dimensions
- The musculoskeletal system has the capacity to adapt in response to changes in the physical environment
- Musculoskeletal adaptation is dependent on *mechanotransduction*: a physiological process by which the myocytes and fibroblasts convert mechanical signals into biological processes
- All musculoskeletal tissues can undergo adaptive change associated with mechanotransduction
- In immobilization and remobilization adaption can be seen in all musculoskeletal tissue
- Adaptive processes are driven by the individual's actions within their environment
- Do not lose sight of the person for the mechanocytes

REFERENCES

1. Sadoshima J-I, Seigo I. Mechanical stretch rapidly activates multiple signal tranduction pathways in cardiac myocytes: potential involvement of an autocrine/paracrine mechanism. EMBO J 1993;12(4):1681–92.
2. Goldspink G. Changes in muscle mass and phenotype and the expression of autocrine and systemic growth factors by muscle in response to stretch and overload. J Anat 1999;194 (Pt 3):323–34.
3. Goldspink G, Yang SY. Effects of activity on growth factor expression. Int J Sport Nutr Exerc Metab 2001;11(Suppl):S21–27.
4. Goldspink G, Williams P, Simpson H. Gene expression in response to muscle stretch. Clin Orthop 2002;403(Suppl):S146–52.
5. Goldspink G. Gene expression in skeletal muscle. Biochem Soc Trans 2002;30(2):285–90.
6. Zeichen J, van Griensven M, Bosch U. The proliferative response of isolated human tendon fibroblasts to cyclic biaxial mechanical strain. Am J Sports Med 2000;28(6):888–92.
7. Graf R, Freyberg M, Kaiser D, et al. Mechanosensitive induction of apoptosis in fibroblasts is regulated by thrombospondin-1 and integrin associated protein (CD47). Apoptosis 2002;7(6):493–8.

8. Eastwood M, Mudera VC, McGrouther DA, et al. Effect of precise mechanical loading on fibroblast populated collagen lattices: morphological changes. Cell Motil Cytoskeleton 1998;40(1):13–21.

9. Grinnell F. Fibroblast–collagen–matrix contraction: growth-factor signalling and mechanical loading. Trends Cell Biol 2000;10(9):362–5.

10. Parsons M, Kessler E, Laurent GJ, et al. Mechanical load enhances procollagen processing in dermal fibroblasts by regulating levels of procollagen C-proteinase. Exp Cell Res 1999;252(2):319–31.

11. Prajapati RT, Chavally-Mis B, Herbage D, et al. Mechanical loading regulates protease production by fibroblasts in three-dimensional collagen substrates. Wound Repair Regen 2000;8(3):226–37.

12. Bosch U, Zeichen J, Skutek M, et al. Effect of cyclical stretch on matrix synthesis of human patellar tendon cells. Unfallchirurg 2002;105(5):437–42.

13. Yamaguchi N, Chiba M, Mitani H. The induction of c-fos mRNA expression by mechanical stress in human periodontal ligament cells. Arch Oral Biol 2002;47(6):465–71.

14. Grinnell F, Ho CH. Transforming growth factor beta stimulates fibroblast–collagen matrix contraction by different mechanisms in mechanically loaded and unloaded matrices. Exp Cell Res 2002;273(2):248–55.

15. Yang H, Alnaqeeb M, Simpson H, et al. Changes in muscle fibre type, muscle mass and IGF-I gene expression in rabbit skeletal muscle subjected to stretch. J Anat 1997;190(Pt 4):613–22.

16. Williams PE. Effect of intermittent stretch on immobilised muscle. Ann Rheum Dis 1988;47:1014–16.

17. Nakashima K, Tsuruga E, Hisanaga Y, et al. Stretching stimulates fibulin-5 expression and controls microfibril bundles in human periodontal ligament cells. J Periodontal Res 2009;44(5):622–7.

18. Burd NA, Holwerda AM, Selby KC, et al. Resistance exercise volume affects myofibrillar protein synthesis and anabolic signalling molecule phosphorylation in young men. J Physiol 2010;588:3119–30.

19. Vader D, Kabla A, Weitz D, et al. Strain-induced alignment in collagen gels. PLoS One 2009;4(6):e5902.

20. Larsen M, Artym VV, Green JA, et al. The matrix reorganized: extracellular matrix remodeling and integrin signaling. Curr Opin Cell Biol 2006;18(5):463–71.

21. Magnusson SP, Langberg H, Kjaer M. The pathogenesis of tendinopathy: balancing the response to loading. Nat Rev Rheumatol 2010;6(5):262–8.

22. Coutinho EL, Gomes AR, França CN, et al. Effect of passive stretching on the immobilized soleus muscle fiber morphology. Braz J Med Biol Res 2004;37(12):1853–61.

23. Goldspink G, Scutt A, Loughna PT, et al. Gene expression in skeletal muscle in response to stretch and force generation. Am J Physiol 1992;262(3 Pt 2):R356–63.

24. Ko KS, McCulloch CA. Intercellular mechanotransduction: cellular circuits that coordinate tissue responses to mechanical loading. Biochem Biophys Res Commun 2001;285(5):1077–83.

25. Chiquet M, Gelman L, Lutz R, et al. From mechanotransduction to extracellular matrix gene expression in fibroblasts. Biochim Biophys Acta 2009;1793(5):911–20.

26. Goldspink G, Tabary C, Tabary J, et al. Effect of denervation on the adaptation of sarcomere number and muscle extensibility to the functional length of the muscle. J Physiol 2009;236(3):733–42.

27. Williams PE, Goldspink G. The effect of denervation and dystrophy on the adaptation of sarcomere number to the functional length of the muscle in young and adult mice. J Anat 1976;122(Pt 2):455–65.

28. Neidlinger-Wilke C, Grood E, Claes L, et al. Fibroblast orientation to stretch begins within three hours. J Orthop Res 2002;20(5):953–6.

29. Akeson WH. An experimental study of joint stiffness. J Bone Joint Surg Am 1961;43:1022–34.

30. Guilak F, Alexopoulos LG, Upton ML, et al. The pericellular matrix as a transducer of bio-mechanical and biochemical signals in articular cartilage. Ann N Y Acad Sci 2006;1068:498–512.
31. MacKenna D, Summerour SR, Villarreal FJ. Role of mechanical factors in modulating cardiac fibroblast function and extracellular matrix synthesis. Cardiovasc Res 2000;46:257–63.
32. Nguyen TD, Liang R, Woo SL, et al. Effects of cell seeding and cyclic stretch on the fiber remodeling in an extracellular matrix-derived bioscaffold. Tissue Eng Part A 2009;15(4):957–63.
33. Balestrini JL, Billiar KL. Magnitude and duration of stretch modulate fibroblast remodeling. J Biomech Eng 2009;131(5):051005.
34. Woo SL, Ritter MA, Amiel D, et al. The biomechanical and biochemical properties of swine tendons: long term effects of exercise on the digital extensors. Connect Tissue Res 1980;7(3):177–83.
35. Gelberman RH, Amiel D, Gonsalves M, et al. The influence of protected passive mobilization on the healing of flexor tendons: a biochemical and microangiographic study. Hand 1981;13(2):120–8.
36. Viidik A, Danielsen C, Oxlund H. On fundamental and phenomenological models, structure and mechanical properties of collagen, elastin and glycosaminoglycan complex. Biorheology 1982;19:437–51.
37. Woo SL, Gomez MA, Sites TJ, et al. The biomechanical and morphological changes in the medial collateral ligament of the rabbit after immobilization and remobilization. J Bone Joint Surg Am 1987;69(8):1200–11.
38. Amiel D, Woo SL-Y, Harwood F, et al. The effect of immobilization on collagen turnover in connective tissue: a biochemical–biomechanical correlation. Acta Orthop Scand 1982;53:325–32.
39. Trudel G, Uhthoff HK. Contractures secondary to immobility: is the restriction articular or muscular? An experimental longitudinal study in the rat knee. Arch Phys Med Rehabil 2000;81(1):6–13.
40. Trudel G, Seki M, Uhthoff HK. Synovial adhesions are more important than pannus prolif-eration in the pathogenesis of knee joint contracture after immobilization: an experimental investigation in the rat. J Rheumatol 2000;27(2):351–7.
41. Trudel G, Jabi M, Uhthoff HK. Localized and adaptive synoviocyte proliferation characteris-tics in rat knee joint contractures secondary to immobility. Arch Phys Med Rehabil 2003;84(9):1350–6.
42. Ando A, Hagiwara Y, Onoda Y, et al. Distribution of type A and B synoviocytes in the adhe-sive and shortened synovial membrane during immobilization of the knee joint in rats. Tohoku J Exp Med 2010;221(2):161–8.
43. Matsumoto F, Trudel G, Uhthoff HK. High collagen type I and low collagen type III levels in knee joint contracture: an immunohistochemical study with histological correlate. Acta Orthop Scand 2002;73(3):335–43.
44. Schollmeier G, Uhthoff HK, Sarkar K, et al. Effects of immobilization on the capsule of the canine glenohumeral joint: a structural functional study. Clin Orthop Relat Res 1994;304:37–42.
45. Schollmeier G, Sarkar K, Fukuhara K, et al. Structural and functional changes in the canine shoulder after cessation of immobilization. Clin Orthop Relat Res 1996;323:310–15.
46. Newton PO, Woo SL, MacKenna DA, et al. Immobilization of the knee joint alters the mechanical and ultrastructural properties of the rabbit anterior cruciate ligament. J Orthop Res 1995;13(2):191–200.
47. Harwood FL, Amiel D. Differential metabolic responses of periarticular ligaments and tendons to joint immobilization. Am Physiol Soc 1990;72(5):1687–91.
48. Onambele GL, Narici MV, Maganaris CN, et al. Calf muscle–tendon properties and postural balance in old age. J Appl Physiol 2006;100:2048–56.

49. Reeves ND, Narici MV, Maganaris CN. Strength training alters the viscoelastic properties of tendons in elderly humans. Muscle Nerve 2003;28:74–81.

50. Reeves ND, Maganaris CN, Ferretti G, et al. Influence of 90-day simulated microgravity on human tendon mechanical properties and the effect of resistive countermeasures. J Appl Physiol 2005;98:2278–86.

51. Noyes FR, Torvik PJ, Hyde WB, et al. Biomechanics of ligament failure. II. An analysis of immobilization, exercise, and reconditioning effects in primates. J Bone Joint Surg Am 1974;56(7):1406–18.

52. Fishkin Z, Miller D, Ritter C, et al. Changes in human knee ligament stiffness secondary to osteoarthritis. J Orthop Res 2002;20(2):204–7.

53. Brage ME, Draganich LF, Pottenger LA, et al. Knee laxity in symptomatic osteoarthritis. Clin Orthop Relat Res 1994;304:184–9.

54. Williams PE, Goldspink G. Changes in sarcomere length and physiological properties in immobilized muscle. J Anat 1978;127(Pt 3):459–68.

55. Tamai K, Kurokawa T, Matsubara I. In situ observation of adjustment of sarcomere length in skeletal muscle under sustained stretch. Nippon Seikeigeka Gakkai Zasshi 1989;63(12): 1558–63.

56. Tabary JC, Tabary C, Tardieu C, et al. Physiological and structural changes in the cat's soleus muscle due to immobilization at different lengths by plaster casts. J Physiol 1972;224(1): 231–44.

57. Tabary JC, Tardieu C, Tardieu G, et al. Experimental rapid sarcomere loss with concomitant hypoextensibility. Muscle Nerve 1981;4(3):198–203.

58. Hayat A, Tardieu C, Tabary JC, et al. Effects of denervation on the reduction of sarcomere number in cat soleus muscle immobilized in shortened position during seven days. J Physiol (Paris) 1978;74(6):563–7.

59. Heslinga JW, Huijing PA. Muscle length–force characteristics in relation to muscle architecture: a bilateral study of gastrocnemius medialis muscles of unilaterally immobilized rats. Eur J Appl Physiol Occup Physiol 1993;66(4):289–98.

60. Heslinga JW, te Kronnie G, Huijing PA. Growth and immobilization effects on sarcomeres: a comparison between gastrocnemius and soleus muscles of the adult rat. Eur J Appl Physiol Occup Physiol 1995;70(1):49–57.

61. Pontén E, Fridén J. Immobilization of the rabbit tibialis anterior muscle in a lengthened position causes addition of sarcomeres in series and extra-cellular matrix proliferation. J Biomech 2008;41(8):1801–4.

62. Herbert RD, Balnave RJ. The effect of position of immobilisation on resting length, resting stiffness, and weight of the soleus muscle of the rabbit. J Orthop Res 1993;11(3):358–66.

63. Matano T, Tamai K, Kurokawa T. Adaptation of skeletal muscle in limb lengthening: a light diffraction study of the sarcomere length in situ. J Orthop Res 1994;12(2):193–6.

64. Scott AB. Change of eye muscle sarcomeres according to eye position. J Pediatr Ophthalmol Strabismus 1994;31(2):85–8.

65. Williams P, Watt P, Bicik V, et al. Effect of stretch combined with electrical stimulation on the type of sarcomeres produced at the ends of muscle fibers. Exp Neurol 1986;93(3):500–9.

66. Williams PE, Goldspink G. Connective tissue changes in immobilised muscle. J Anat 1984;138(2):343–50.

67. Williams P, Kyberd P, Simpson H, et al. The morphological basis of increased stiffness of rabbit tibialis anterior during surgical limb-lengthening. J Anat 1998;193:131–8.

68. Williams PE, Catanese T, Lucey EG, et al. The importance of stretch and contractile activity in the prevention of connective tissue accumulation in muscle. J Anat 1988;158:109–14.

69. Savio SL-Y, Gelberman RH, Cobb NG, et al. The importance of controlled passive mobilization on flexor tendon healing. Acta Orthop Scand 1981;52(6):615–22.

70. Evans EB, Eggers GWN, Butler JK, et al. Experimental immobilisation and remobilisation of rat knee joints. J Bone Joint Surg 1960;42A(5):737–58.

71. Madden JW, Peacock EE. Studies on the biology of collagen during wound healing. I. Rate of collagen synthesis and deposition in cutaneous wounds of the rat. Surgery 1968;64(1):288–94.

72. Madden JW, Peacock EE. Studies on the biology of collagen during wound healing. III. Dynamic metabolism of scar collagen and remodelling of dermal wounds. Ann Surg 1971;174:511–20.

73. Madden JW, DeVore G, Arem AJ. A rational postoperative management program for metacarpophalangeal joint implant arthroplasty. J Hand Surg 1977;2:358–66.

74. Hunt TK, Van Winkle W. Normal repair. In: Hunt TK, Dunphy JE, editors. Fundamentals of wound management. New York: Appleton-Century-Crofts; 1979:2–67.

75. Baur PS, Parks DH. The myofibroblast anchoring strand: the fibronectin connection in wound healing and possible loci of collagen fibril assembly. J Trauma 1983;23:853–62.

76. Tillman LJ, Cummings GS. Biology mechanisms of connective tissue mutability. In: Currier DP, Nelson RM, editors. Dynamics of human biological tissue. Philadelphia: FA Davies; 1993:1–44.

77. Strickland JW, Glogovac V. Digital function following flexor tendon repair in zone 2: a comparison of immobilization and controlled passive motion techniques. J Hand Surg 1980;5(6):537–43.

78. Fronek J, Frank C, Amiel D, et al. The effect of intermittent passive motion (IMP) in the healing of medial collateral ligament. Proc Orthop Res Soc 1983;8:31.

79. Vailas AC, Tipton CM, Matthes RD, et al. Physical activity and its influence on the repair process of medial collateral ligament. Connect Tissue Res 1981;9:25–31.

80. Loitz BJ, Zernicke RF, Vailas AC, et al. Effects of short-term immobilization versus continuous passive motion on the biomechanical and biochemical properties of the rabbit tendon. Clin Orthop 1989;244:265–71.

81. Pneumaticos SG, McGarvey WC, Mody DR, et al. The effects of early mobilization in the healing of achilles tendon repair. Foot Ankle Int 2000;21(7):551–7.

82. Sanders JE, Goldstein BS. Collagen fibril diameters increase and fibril densities decrease in skin subjected to repetitive compressive and shear stresses. J Biomech 2001;34(12):1581–7.

83. Balestrini JL, Billiar KL. Equibiaxial cyclic stretch stimulates fibroblasts to rapidly remodel fibrin. J Biomech 2006;39(16):2983–90.

84. Noyes FR. Functional properties of knee ligaments and alterations induced by immobilization: a correlative biomechanical and histological study in primates. Clin Orthop Relat Res 1977;123:210–42.

85. Riley DA, Van Dyke JM. The effects of active and passive stretching on muscle length. Phys Med Rehabil Clin North Am 2012;23(1):51–7.

86. Aquino CF, Fonseca ST, Gonçalves GG, et al. Stretching versus strength training in lengthened position in subjects with tight hamstring muscles: a randomized controlled trial. Man Ther 2009;15(1):26–31.

87. Bamman MM, Shipp JR, Jiang J, et al. Mechanical load increases muscle IGF-I and androgen receptor mRNA concentrations in humans. Am J Physiol Endocrinol Metab 2001;280(3):E383–90.

88. McKoy G, Ashley W, Mander J, et al. Expression of insulin growth factor-1 splice variants and structural genes in rabbit skeletal muscle induced by stretch and stimulation. J Physiol 1999;516(Pt 2):583–92.

89. Baldwin KM, Haddad F. Skeletal muscle plasticity: cellular and molecular responses to altered physical activity paradigms. Am J Phys Med Rehabil 2002;81(11 Suppl):S40–51.

90. Palmar RM, Reeds PJ, Lobley GE, et al. The effect of intermittent changes in tension on protein and collagen synthesis in isolated rabbit muscle. Biomech J 1981;198:491–98.

91. Loughna PT, Morgan MJ. Passive stretch modulates denervation induced alterations in skeletal muscle myosin heavy chain mRNA levels. Pflugers Arch 1999;439(1–2):52–5.

92. Loughna P, Goldspink G, Goldspink DF. Effect of inactivity and passive stretch on protein turnover in phasic and postural rat muscles. J Appl Physiol 1986;61(1):173–9.

93. Krishnan L, Underwood CJ, Maas S, et al. Effect of mechanical boundary conditions on orientation of angiogenic microvessels. Cardiovasc Res 2008;78(2):324–32.

94. Vernon RB, Angello JC, Iruela-Arispe ML, et al. Reorganization of basement membrane matrices by cellular traction promotes the formation of cellular networks in vitro. Lab Invest 1992;66(5):536–47.

95. Lee RT. Lessons from lymph: flow-guided vessel formation. Circ Res 2003;92(7):701–3.

96. Gelberman RH, Menon J, Gonsalves M, et al. The effects of mobilization on the vascularization of healing flexor tendons in dogs. Clin Orthop Relat Res 1980;153:283–9.

97. DeFeudis FV, DeFeudis PAF. Elements of the behavioral code. London: Academic Press; 1977.

98. Kidd G, Lawes N, Musa I. Understanding neuromuscular plasticity: a basis for clinical rehabilitation. London: Edward Arnold; 1992.

99. Lederman E. Neuromuscular rehabilitation in manual and physical therapies. Edinburgh: Elsevier; 2010.

100. de Jong BM, Coert JH, Stenekes MW, et al. Cerebral reorganisation of human hand movement following dynamic immobilisation. Neuroreport 2003;14(13):1693–6.

101. Patten C, Kamen G. Adaptations in motor unit discharge activity with force control training in young and older human adults. Eur J Appl Physiol 2000;83(2–3):128–43.

102. Kaneko F, Murakami T, Onari K, et al. Decreased cortical excitability during motor imagery after disuse of an upper limb in humans. Clin Neurophysiol 2003;114(12):2397–403.

103. Liepert J, Tegenthoff M, Malin JP. Changes of cortical motor area size during immobilization. Electroenceph Clin Neurophysiol 1995;97:382–6.

104. Seki K, Taniguchi Y, Narusawa M. Effects of joint immobilization on firing rate modulation of human motor units. J Physiol 2001;530(3):507–19.

CHAPTER 5

Specificity in ROM Rehabilitation

Often individuals (as well as animals) overcome their injury and range of movement (ROM) losses by taking actions that resemble the movement patterns which they have lost: a person with a sprained ankle will attempt to gradually walk; a tennis player with a shoulder injury will attempt to gradually return to playing tennis. Similarly a patient with a frozen shoulder, given time and without any rehabilitation, will often regain their full ROM by daily use of their shoulder.[1] This behaviour can be considered to be Nature's "gold standard" for movement recovery – *practise what you aim to recover*.

However, in physical therapy we provide a curious management. Patients are often given exercise that has no resemblance to the movements that they wish to recover. This raises the possibility that what is prescribed in clinic may not provide the most effective ROM rehabilitation. For example, would floor exercise or manual stretching of the hip improve stride length?

This chapter will explore the following topics:

- Can commonly prescribed stretching exercise improve functional activities?
- Can manual stretching techniques improve functional activities?
- What kind of gain is expected to carry over from the ROM challenge to functional activities?
- How close to the goal task does the ROM challenge have to be?
- What factors can improve the carry-over between ROM exercise and functional activities?

SPECIFICITY AND GENERALIZATION

In order to understand how to transform clinical gain into functional improvement we need to look at the specificity phenomenon in adaptation.

When we learn a new skill the motor, tissue and physiological adaptation is specific to that particular task (*specificity*).[2–8] This allows the task to be optimally performed with minimal energy expenditure, physical stress and error. This adaptation is unique, and optimized for that particular activity, but may be unsuitable for a different activity.[9–12] This is why the performance of cross country skiing does not improve by dancing practice.[13] However, if specificity in adaptation was absolute it would mean that we would have to learn the task as well as each of its infinite variations. This problem in adaptation is overcome by our ability to carry-over learning or training experiences to variations of *the same* activity/task (*generalization*). So once a movement has been learned it can be performed with many variations without having to practise them all.[14–17] Hence, throwing a ball can be performed in conditions that have never been encountered during the training. Similarly, we can drive an unfamiliar hired car without having to re-learn driving.

The generalization–specificity principle in learning and training has important implications for therapeutic stretching. In many stretching approaches it is expected that particular techniques or exercise will help to improve a wide range of functional activities. An example is core stability exercise in which specific trunk muscle training is believed to enhance performance in many different sports and daily activities. Similarly, there is a common expectation that stretching techniques would improve a variety of daily activities. For example, muscle energy technique (MET) applied to shoulder extensors would be expected to improve many functional overhead tasks.

On the other hand, specificity implies that the treatment has to closely resemble the goal activity,[18,19] i.e. walking should be rehabilitated by walking, standing by standing and balance by balancing. Equally, ROM challenges should replicate closely the movements being recovered; for example, shoulder ROM should be challenged during functional overhead activities (Fig. 5.1). Specificity implies that, if the stretching and goals of rehabilitation are dissimilar, there would be an ineffective carry-over of clinical gains to functional improvements. For example, it would be expected that MET of shoulder extensors would be ineffective in improving functional overhead activities. This is because there is no resemblance between the muscle recruitment sequences during MET and those of a functional movement such as reaching overhead.

From a therapeutic perspective, a generalization principle is very attractive and therefore prevalent in physical therapies; all that is needed is a particular set of universal exercises to improve a wide spectrum of daily activities. On the other hand, a specificity principle means that treatment has to focus on a wider selection of affected activities. The specificity–generalization issue is not well researched in physical therapies, and for answers we need to look at motor learning and training principles, in particular at the transfer principle in training.

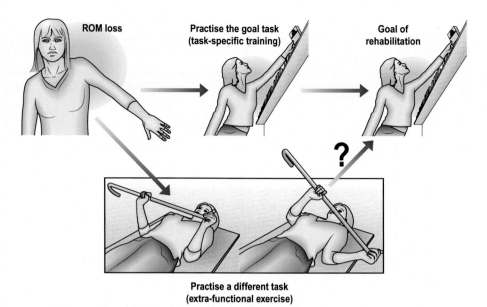

ROM loss

Practise the goal task
(task-specific training)

Goal of
rehabilitation

?

Practise a different task
(extra-functional exercise)

FIGURE 5.1 Range of movement (ROM) rehabilitation: task specific or extra-functional training? Movement rehabilitation often uses exercises that are dissimilar to the goal task, rather than using the task itself. There is an assumption that something special is happening in the extra-functional but not the specific task training.

Transfer of training

Imagine a clinical situation in which a patient with flexion contracture of the hip is given particular exercises to recover hip ROM; say, kneeling on all-fours quads stretch. The ultimate aim is to influence hip function during walking rather than improve the performance of this particular exercise. By prescribing such exercises we assume that there are some elements within the exercise that would generalize and carry-over to improve walking. This carry-over is called *transfer*; it is how the performance of a particular task (say, walking) is influenced by practise of another activity (quads stretch exercise).[10,20–22]

In physical therapies it is often *assumed* that several elements can be transferred between the exercise and the goal task; using hip exercise as an example (Fig. 5.2):

- **Recruitment sequences** – One common assumption is that particular recruitment sequences, such as relative on–off timing and duration of hip synergists, would transfer from the exercise to the task.
- **Task parameters** – Another assumption is that transfer could be one or several of the task parameters such as the force, velocity, range and endurance of hip muscles.

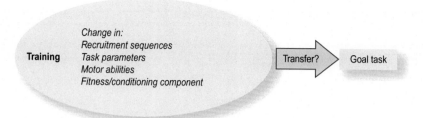

FIGURE 5.2 The content of transfer. There is a widely held assumption in physical therapies that all these elements can be transferred between different tasks.

- **Motor abilities** – Motor abilities are movement traits of an individual that underlie skilled performance. There is a common belief that particular motor abilities, such as balance or coordination, could transfer between tasks. For example, hip coordination during walking would be normalized by improving trunk–pelvic–hip coordination exercise on the floor. Or, that balancing on a Swiss ball would transfer to improvements in balance during walking.
- **Fitness/conditioning component** – Another possibility is that the exercise could improve some localized atrophy or general fitness. This conditioning effect could carry-over to improve the target skill. For example, the all-fours hip extension exercise would help recover some of the extensor muscle wasting in the affected limb and therefore improve hip extension during walking.

The question that emerges is which of these movement elements can transfer between the exercise and the goal task? To answer this we need to look at the distance which the movement elements have to carry over, i.e. how close is training to its goals.

Measuring similarities

To explore resemblance we need some form of yard-stick to "measure" this distance. This can be assessed by looking at whether the training is within the same task (*within-task*), e.g. train in walking to improve walking, or between two dissimilar tasks *(between-task)*, e.g. training on all fours to improve walking.

An example of exercise that aims to utilize within-task transfer is the common use of weights during walking or running. Here, the training and the task resemble each other but with the added overloading of force. Within-task transfer is represented in ROM rehabilitation by the expectation that improvement of force in one range would carry over to other, unpractised ranges.

Between-task training aims to improve a particular task by training or treating in a different task; for example, the common practice of balancing on a Swiss ball in order to improve balance during walking. Here, the focus is on balance transfer but the exercise is dissimilar to the goal task (walking). Another example would be to train for explosive force by vertical jumps (one task), but with the aim of improving sprinting (another task), an activity that also requires an explosive force. Between-task transfer is represented in ROM rehabilitation by the expectation that practising the all-fours hip extension exercise on the floor would improve walking hip ROM.

A further measure of resemblance is *similarity* and *dissimilarity* of the movement patterns between the exercise and the target task.[23,24] For example, does the movement of the leg during all-fours leg extension exercise resemble the movement patterns of the leg during walking?

Whether the training is within-task or similar provides four categories for assessing the "distance" between the ROM challenges and the goals of rehabilitation. The challenges can be (Fig. 5.3):

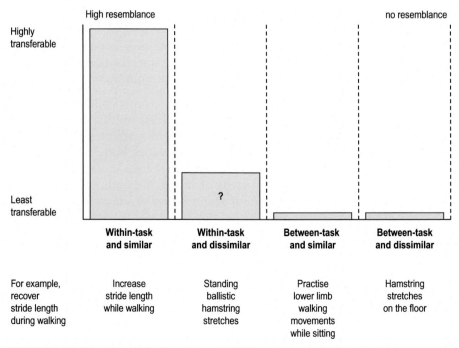

FIGURE 5.3 Assessing similarity and transferability between the training and the rehabilitation goals.

A. Within-task:
- Within-task-similar
- Within-task-dissimilar

B. Between-task:
- Between-task-similar
- Between-task-dissimilar

Imagine again the patient who has reduced hip extension that limits walking. The training would be *within-task-similar* if the person is instructed simply to walk with a wider stride. Another possibility is to walk while performing pelvis-stabilizing exercises. In this case, the movement is within the task of walking but is somewhat dissimilar to it *(within-task-dissimilar)*. Performing leg movements that resemble walking while sitting would be an example of an exercise which is *between-task-similar*. The rehabilitation would be *between-task* and *dissimilar* to walking if the patient is instructed to perform a hip extension exercise while lying prone.

Now that we have a way of measuring resemblance we can explore in which of these categories transfer is most likely to occur.

STUDIES OF SPECIFICITY AND TRANSFER

Overall, several decades of studies in motor learning suggest that specificity is the dominant outcome of training/practice and transfer between tasks is mostly absent and if present is considered to be insignificant.[25-32]

Specificity in movement can already be observed in young children.[5] It seems that each task in their movement repertoire is learned specifically, with little or no transfer between tasks that share the same motor abilities. For example, dynamic balance skills do not transfer to static balance skills and vice versa. A high level of fine motor control in the hand may help in drawing but not in playing with Lego bricks, an activity that also depends on fine motor control. This lack of transfer of motor abilities between tasks has also been shown in adults.[25,33]

Some within-task transfer has been shown in sports training but it tends to be modest and unpredictable. Sprinting performance was shown to improve by single-leg horizontal jumps but not by vertical jumps using both limbs, such as jump squats.[18] Transfer may fail to occur even in trainings that seem to closely resemble the task. For example, resistance sprint training using a towing device fails to improve sprint performance.[34] Similarly, off-ice skating exercises do not improve on-ice performance in speed skaters.[35] Even activities that look identical, such as sprinting and endurance running, each have their unique, non-transferable knee force–angle profiles. This specificity is also observed anatomically. The fascicle length of leg muscles is greater in sprinters than in distance runners.[36,37] That is why marathon runners are not great sprinters, although the movements they perform in running look very similar.

Even in within-task training some elements of the task parameters may not transfer well. For example, the gains of resistance training at one speed may not transfer well to another speed of the same movement.[38-41] Strength gains are greatest at the training velocity with some carry-over to other velocities.[42] Similarly, strength gains are greatest at the training angles with some transfer to other ranges (see more below).[43-45]

There is substantial evidence demonstrating that between-task training gains do not transfer well. Core stability exercises fail to improve sports performance (between-task-dissimilar).[46-48] Different forms of resistance exercise have failed to improve specific sports activities such as football kicks, sprinting, netball, hockey, throwing velocity in water polo and rowing.[18,49-55] Even resistance training in one particular posture may not transfer strength gains to other postures.[56]

In elite gymnasts, athletes, judo competitors and dancers, training to hold difficult, sport-specific postures does not transfer balance ability to commonly used unspecific standing postures.[57-60] Cross-training by cycling does not improve running and may even reduce running economy.[61-63] Training in isolated tasks, such as hip flexibility or trunk-strengthening activities, does not improve the economy of walking or running.[64] Vertical jumps are improved by training in vertical but not by training in sideways jumps.[65] Upper limb resistance exercises do not improve arm coordination,[66] and so on.

All these studies provide a very clear message: the greater the distance in resemblance the less likely is the transfer. Optimal training gains occur when the training is within-task and similar to its goals. Least effective are between-task and dissimilar training. But what about stretching? How likely is it to provide performance gains?

Transfer in stretching

Most traditional stretching exercises represent training which is between-tasks and dissimilar to its goals (Ch. 1). Hence, we would not expect transfer to occur. Indeed, regular and warm-up stretching, in all its variations, has failed to demonstrate transfer of gains to sports performance.[67-69] One study demonstrated that 4 weeks of contract–relax stretch training (proprioceptive neuromuscular facilitation) of the knee improved flexion range but did not alter the active movement performance (peak isokinetic quadriceps torque).[70] In another study, 10 weeks of lower limb stretching had no effect on vertical jumps.[71] Similarly, 6 weeks of passive static stretching and contract–relax stretching improved the ROM but neither had any significant effect on the drop jumps.[72] In contrast, one study has shown that 8 weeks of upper limb passive stretching was shown to improve bench presses.[73] However, a recent review found no benefit in acute bouts of static stretching for any form of muscular performance.[69]

These studies suggest that traditional, extra-functional stretching approaches are unlikely to provide performance gain because of their dissimilarity to the goal task. But what about ROM challenges that are within-task? Is generalization possible? Would an improvement in shoulder control of 0–90° flexion improve the control of other ranges, say, 90–120°? Or would improvements in reaching range in the frontal plane be generalized to improvement of the same movement but in the coronal plane?

Motor learning studies suggest that learning a task in one range can generalize/ transfer to other angles of the same task. This was demonstrated in a study in which subjects had to catch a series of light and heavy balls with either a "bent" or a "straight" arm configuration.[32] It was found that the learning of catching in one configuration transferred 100% to the other. Here, the contents of transfer are the recruitment sequences of the movement (see Transfer of Training). Force training in one range seems to be angle/ROM specific.[43-45] However, there may be some carry-over of force gains to other untrained angles,[42] in particular if the full range is practised rather than specific angles.[29,31]

In summary, optimal transfer and generalization occur when the ROM challenges are within-task and similar to the movement goals. The four movement parameters, force, range, speed and endurance, are the most likely elements to be transferred or generalized during task-specific training.

STUDIES OF SPECIFICITY AND TRANSFER IN PATIENTS

So far this chapter has explored the specificity in healthy individuals. The question that remains is whether adaptation principles apply to individuals with pathological ROM losses. In a limited number of studies transfer of rehabilitation gains has been examined in patients with musculoskeletal injuries and pain conditions and in patients with central nervous system damage.

In individuals suffering from chronic neck pain, extra-functional neck exercises do not transfer to improvement in functional head–neck movements (between-tasks and dissimilar).[74] In contrast, a positive transfer of postural stability was demonstrated in a study of balance in subjects with lateral ankle sprain. Training under moderately unstable conditions transferred to improvements in postural control under more challenging stability conditions (within-task-similar).[75] However, we do not know whether these improvements would transfer to functional activities outside the research lab.

For stroke patients resistance cycling or seated strength exercise improves strength in these activities but has little or no effect on walking;[76,77] sitting and reaching training improves sitting and reaching and the production of vertical force through the leg as they lean forward.[78] The vertical force improvement in the leg seems to transfer to improvement in getting up from sitting, but nothing from that training transfers to walking. However, training of stroke patients in walking improves walking speed and distance but not balance.[79–81] Balance seems to be improved by challenging balance.[82,83] But challenging static balance in standing might not transfer well to dynamic balance during walking.[84] So here, too, transfer can be unpredictable and finicky.

Studies of individuals with age-related or pathological ROM losses suggest a lack of transfer between tasks. One study of postmenopausal women found no effect of regular exercise and stretching on walking performance.[85] In one study of older individuals with hip flexor contracture, 8 weeks of hip and ankle stretching provided a modest improvement in passive ROM (hip 6.8°, ankle 3.5°) but failed to improve stride length.[86] In a similar study, 10 weeks of hip and ankle stretching improved hip flexibility (1.5°) but failed to show significant improvements in gait performance. Twelve weeks of foot exercise that included ankle stretching failed to improve physical gait performance in elderly individuals.[87] In a recent study passive stretching was shown to increase passive hip ROM (5°) and stride length (by 2.7 cm) during comfortable but not during fast walking speeds.[88] However, at neither walking speed was there any improvement in peak hip extension or peak anterior pelvic tilt, i.e. there was no transfer of hip flexibility from the exercise to the walking.[89,90] This is likely to be due to the failure to emulate the complex intermuscular coordination of the hip during walking by passive stretching (Ch. 8). It would have been useful in all these studies to include a task-specific group that trained in walking faster or with a wider gait.

In 2011, a Cochrane systematic review reported that various forms of traditional stretching for contractures failed to improve functional activities.[91]

IMPLICATIONS FOR ROM REHABILITATION

From the evidence discussed above there is a strong case for recommending training, exercise and treatment approaches that are task-specific and similar to the rehabilitation goals,[26,92] i.e. walking rehabilitates walking. It seems that the various contents of transfer may be generalized but only when they are practised within the same task (within-task and similar).[17,93–96]

Table 5.1 Transferability in range of movement (ROM) challenges. Functional approaches resemble normal daily activities and are therefore more likely to transfer benefits to the tasks which are the goals of rehabilitation. Extra-functional approaches, comprising many traditional stretching methods, are often dissimilar to normal movement and are therefore unlikely to transfer gain to functional tasks

	Management/ROM challenge	Does it resemble functional tasks?	
Functional	Recovery behaviour	**Yes**	Most transferable
	Managed recovery behaviour	**Yes**	
	Assisted recovery behaviour (functional stretching)	**Yes**	
Extra-functional	Ballistic stretching	No	
	Dynamic stretching	No (not often)	
	Muscle energy technique	No	
	Passive stretching	No	
	Spinal manipulation	No	
	Traction	No	
	Articulation	No	
	Harmonic	No	
	Strain counterstrain	No	
	Cranial	No	Least transferable

The specificity principle suggests that ROM rehabilitation should be closely tailored to the individual's movement repertoire.[92] Hence, ROM rehabilitation of the hip will differ between a footballer and a dancer. Initially, the ROM rehabilitation will aim to recover shared functional activities, such as stride length in walking or climbing stairs. However, at a particular point the rehabilitation would diverge to take into account the individual's unique movement repertoire. Footballers would be rehabilitated with end-ROM challenges during movements that resemble football passes, kicks, etc. Dancers would require end-ROM challenges in sequences that are selected from their dance repertoire (Chs 1 and 12).

At the bottom end of the transferability scale are training/treatments that are extra-functional and dissimilar to the goals of rehabilitation (between-task and dissimilar). Many traditional stretching techniques/exercises are often performed on either the treatment table or the floor and are therefore dissimilar to functional "real-life" movements (Table 5.1). The consequence is motor control and peripheral adaptation that is specific to these clinical practices but that is completely different from the complex intermuscular coordination required during functional activities (Ch. 8).[96] These approaches are unlikely to transfer improvements and may reduce the efficacy of rehabilitation, i.e. floor hip-extension exercise is unlikely to transfer any significant gains to walking. Passive manual stretching approaches will fail to drive any motor control adaptation. They are therefore unlikely to promote any level of generalization or transfer of passive ROM gains into active ones (Ch. 8).

Some patients may be unable to perform task-specific activities because of pain, motor control losses, multiple injuries or simply fear. In these circumstances there may be a place for extra-functional ROM rehabilitation. The rehabilitation could commence on the treatment table or the floor. However, as soon as the patient demonstrates an ability to stand the treatment, should switch to that context level. In situations where deconditioning is present there may be a low-level transfer of the task parameters (force, endurance) to functional activities.[40,97-101] However, this seems to occur only when atrophy reaches a critically low level.[102] Even in these conditions, exercises that challenge the task parameters (force, endurance) and are practised within the goal task seem to provide better functional gains.[92,103-108]

In summary, there is potential for ROM recovery to generalize within a task but transfer is poor between tasks. Even within task-specific training/treatment, the potential and degree of generalization and transfer can be unpredictable. Providing ROM rehabilitation that is task specific is a simple clinical solution to overcome this unpredictability.

PROMOTING GENERALIZATION AND TRANSFER IN ROM REHABILITATION

There are several clinical practices that could help promote generalization during ROM rehabilitation; in particular, the use of variable practice and random scheduling.[25,92,109]

Most functional activities contain numerous variations of particular tasks, and this should be reflected in the rehabilitation. It has been demonstrated that practising variations of a particular task tends to promote within-task generalization. Furthermore, transfer within-task tends to occur more readily when larger movement ranges are used during practice.[94,110] Practising within a narrow range tends to promote control that is more specific to the particular range but reduces the transfer to other ranges.[29,30,43-45,56] Applying these principles to the shoulder, a ROM rehabilitation could include reaching movements performed in a wide range of angles and different movement planes. It should also include variations in force, velocity and fatiguing challenges within a reaching task (see video demonstration).

ROM rehabilitation in one task may not necessarily improve the control in another; each activity has its own unique ROM control profile. Therefore, ROM should be challenged in as many tasks as possible. A reaching movement could be mixed with other tasks such as lifting or pulling movements. Stride length could be challenged during walking, stepping over a high obstacle, stepping onto a high step, etc.

The task variations should be introduced in a random manner.[24,25,111-115] It was found that random training practices provide more effective motor learning and generalization than practices where each skill is performed repeatedly in blocks – *jumbled practices lead to better performance!*

Patients with central nervous system conditions, such as Alzheimer's and Parkinson's disease, may require more simplified scheduling practices.[23] They seem to improve their learning and transfer when the tasks are practised individually and repetitively.[116-118] Clinically, a pragmatic approach is probably useful for scheduling of training/treatment: using the order that the patient can cope with, rather than imposing a strict protocol.

There are other training factors that could help promote generalization, such as performing whole versus fragmented movement and using external versus internal focus of attention. These topics will be discussed further in Chapter 8.[119,120]

A NOTE ON SENSORY SPECIFICITY

When we learn a certain movement it is stored as a unified sensory–motor representation, with each task/activity having a unique sensory–motor signature specific to that task.[12,121-124] How a certain task "feels" is memorized as a reference for future execution of a similar movement.[125,126] This sensory memory provides an error detection system that plays a role in correction of movement and motor learning.[19]

Sensory specificity may play a role in impeding transfer between dissimilar tasks or movement that have been practiced under different sensory conditions.[24,127-134] This was demonstrated in a study in which subjects were trained to walk across a balance beam either with or without vision. It was found that the participants improved their balance more in the sensory condition for which they trained.[128,135] Even learning tactile discrimination of a particular texture may fail to improve tactile discrimination of an unfamiliar texture.[129-131,136] This sensory specificity was demonstrated in blind individuals.[137] They outperformed sighted individuals on palpation tasks that use Braille-like dot patterns (a familiar pattern). However, they did not differ from sighted individuals when presented with a novel palpation discrimination task (a surface with ridges of different widths and orientations).

Sensory specificity suggests that task-specific training creates unique sensory–motor experience that may not transfer to other tasks.[138-142] This means that traditional stretching methods may imprint specific sensory–motor experiences that would not transfer to functional activities (see motor control, Ch. 8).[142]

SUMMARY

- Specificity is the unique motor, muscular and tissue adaptation brought about by exercise/rehabilitation
- Generalization is the ability to carry-over the performance gains in a particular task to variations of the same task
- Transfer is the measure of how the performance of a particular skill is influenced by practice of another activity
- Transfer of training gains is more likely to occur if the ROM challenge resembles the goal activity (within-task and similar)
- Task-specific ROM rehabilitation is likely to be more effective than extra-functional training
- Generalization is more likely to occur in task-specific training
- Performing random variations of the task can facilitate generalization
- ROM challenges that are dissimilar to the goal activities are less likely to transfer gains and should only be used in conditions in which the patient is unable to perform functional activities
- Many traditional stretching approaches, active or passive, are often dissimilar and lack task specificity. They are therefore unlikely to promote functional recovery
- Message to the patient – practise what you aim to recover (a lot)

REFERENCES

1. Diercks RL, Stevens M. Gentle thawing of the frozen shoulder: a prospective study of supervised neglect versus intensive physical therapy in seventy-seven patients with frozen shoulder syndrome followed up for two years. J Shoulder Elbow Surg 2004;13(5):499–502.
2. DeAnna LA, Boychuk J, Remple MS, et al. Motor training induces experience-specific patterns of plasticity across motor cortex and spinal cord. J Appl Physiol 2006;101:1776–82.
3. Millet GP, Vleck VE, Bentley DJ. Physiological differences between cycling and running: lessons from triathletes. Sports Med 2009;39(3):179–206.
4. Withers RT, Sherman WM, Miller JM, et al. Specificity of the anaerobic threshold in endurance trained cyclists and runners. Eur J Appl Physiol Occup Physiol 1981;47(1):93–104.
5. Haga M, Pedersen AV, Sigmundsson H. Interrelationship among selected measures of motor skills. Child Care Health Dev 2008;34(2):245–8.
6. Magel JR, Foglia GF, McArdle WD, et al. Specificity of swim training on maximum oxygen uptake. J Appl Physiol 1975;38(1):151–5.
7. Beneke R, Hofmann C, Strauss N, et al. Maximal lactate steady state depends on sports discipline. Med Sci Sports Exerc 1993;25(5):Suppl abstract 365.

8. Town GP, Bradley SS. Maximal metabolic responses of deep and shallow water running in trained runners. Med Sci Sports Exerc 1991;23:238–41.

9. Holding DH. Principles of training. Oxford: Pergamon; 1965.

10. Osgood CE. The similarity paradox in human learning: a resolution. Psychol Rev 1949;56:132–43.

11. van Ingen Schenau GJ, de Koning JJ, de Groot G. Optimisation of sprinting performance in running, cycling and speed skating. Sports Med 1994;17(4):259–75.

12. Henry F. Specificity vs. generality in learning motor skills. In: 61st Annual Proceedings of the College of the Physical Education Association; 1958.

13. Alricsson M, Werner S. The effect of pre-season dance training on physical indices and back pain in elite cross-country skiers: a prospective controlled intervention study. Br J Sports Med 2004;38(2):148–53.

14. Shadmehr R. Generalization as a behavioral window to the neural mechanisms of learning internal models. Hum Mov Sci 2004;23:543–68.

15. Krakauer JW, Mazzoni P, Ghazizadeh A, et al. Generalization of motor learning depends on the history of prior action. PLoS Biol 2006;4(10):e316.

16. Savin DN, Morton SM. Asymmetric generalization between the arm and leg following prism-induced visuomotor adaptation. Exp Brain Res 2008;186(1):175–82.

17. Wilde H, Shea CH. Proportional and nonproportional transfer of movement sequences. Q J Exp Psychol (Hove) 2006;59(9):1626–47.

18. Young WB. Transfer of strength and power training to sports performance. Int J Sports Physiol Perform 2006;1(2):74–83.

19. Lederman E. Neuromuscular rehabilitation in manul and physical therapies. Edinburgh: Elsevier; 2010.

20. Čoh M, Jovanović-Golubović D, Bratić M. Motor learning in sports. Phys Educ Sport 2004;2(1):45–59.

21. Morris SL, Sharpe MH. PNF revisited. Physiother Theory Prac 1993;9:43–51.

22. Cratty BJ. Movement behaviour and motor learning. 2nd ed. London: Henry Kimpton; 1967.

23. Boutin A, Blandin Y. On the cognitive processes underlying contextual interference: contributions of practice schedule, task similarity and amount of practice. Hum Mov Sci 2010;29:910–20.

24. Boutin A, Blandin Y. Cognitive underpinnings of contextual interference during motor learning. Acta Psychol 2010;135:233–9.

25. Schmidt RA, Lee TD. Motor control and learning: a behavioral emphasis. 4th ed. Champaign, IL: Human Kinetics; 2005:271–97, 321–63, 432–59.

26. Healy AF, Wohldmann EL. Specificity effects in training and transfer of speeded responses. J Exp Psychol Learn Mem Cogn 2006;32(3):534–46.

27. Goodbody SJ, Wolpert DM. Temporal and amplitude generalization in motor learning. J Neurophysiol 1998;79:1825–38.

28. Mattar AA, Ostry DJ. Generalization of dynamics learning across changes in movement amplitude. J Neurophysiol 2010;104(1):426–38.

29. Graves JE, Pollock ML, Jones AE, et al. Specificity of limited range of motion variable resistance training. Med Sci Sports Exerc 1989;21(1):84–9.

30. Graves JE, Pollock ML, Leggett SH, et al. Limited range-of-motion lumbar extension strength training. Med Sci Sports Exerc 1992;24(1):128–33.

31. Barak Y, Ayalon M, Dvir Z. Transferability of strength gains from limited to full range of motion. Med Sci Sports Exerc 2004;36(8):1413–20.

32. Morton SM, Lang CE, Bastian AJ. Inter- and intra-limb generalization of adaptation during catching. Exp Brain Res 2001;141(4):438–45.

33. Fleishman EA. An analysis of positioning movements and static reactions. J Exp Psychol 1958;55:213–46.

34. Kristensen GO, van den Tillaar R, Ettema GJ. Velocity specificity in early-phase sprint training. J Strength Cond Res 2006;20(4):833–7.

35. de Boer RW, Ettema GJ, Faessen BG, et al. Specific characteristics of speed skating: implications for summer training. Med Sci Sports Exerc 1987;19(5):504–10.

36. Shealy MJ, Callister R, Dudley GA, et al.. Human torque velocity adaptations to sprint, endurance, or combined modes of training. Am J Sports Med 1992;20(5):581–6.

37. Abe T, Kumagai K, Brechue WF. Fascicle length of leg muscles is greater in sprinters than distance runners. Med Sci Sports Exerc 2000;32(6):1125–9.

38. Ingebrigtsen J, Holtermann A, Roeleveld K. Effects of load and contraction velocity during three-week biceps curls training on isometric and isokinetic performance. J Strength Cond Res 2009;23(6):1670–6.

39. Blazevich AJ, Jenkins D. Physical performance differences between weight-trained sprinters and weight trainers. J Sci Med Sport 1998;1(1):12–21.

40. Frontera WR, Meredith CN, O'Reilly KP, et al. Strength conditioning in older men: skeletal muscle hypertrophy and improved function. J Appl Physiol 1988;64:1038–44.

41. Pereira MIR, Gomes PSC. Movement velocity in resistance training. Sports Med 2003;33(6):427–38.

42. Morrissey MC, Harman EA, Johnson MJ. Resistance training modes: specificity and effectiveness. Med Sci Sports Exerc 1988;27(1995):648–60.

43. Folland JP, Hawker K, Leach B, et al. Strength training: isometric training at a range of joint angles versus dynamic training. J Sports Sci 2005;23(8):817–24.

44. Weir JP, Housh DJ, Housh TJ, et al. The effect of unilateral eccentric weight training and detraining on joint angle specificity, cross-training, and the bilateral task deficit. J Orthop Sports Phys Ther 1995;22(5):207–15.

45. Weir JP, Housh TJ, Weir LL, et al. Effects of unilateral isometric strength training on joint angle specificity and cross-training. Eur J Appl Physiol Occup Physiol 1995;70(4):337–43.

46. Hibbs AE, Thompson KG, French D, et al. Optimizing performance by improving core stability and core strength. Sports Med 2008;38(12):995–1008.

47. Parkhouse KL, Ball N. Influence of dynamic versus static core exercises on performance in field based fitness tests. J Bodyw Mov Ther 2011;15(4):517–24.

48. Okada T, Huxel KC, Nesser TW. Relationship between core stability, functional movement, and performance. J Strength Cond Res 2011;25(1):252–61.

49. Aagaard P, Simonsen EB, Trolle M, et al. Specificity of training velocity and training load on gains in isokinetic knee joint strength. Acta Physiol Scand 1996;156(2):123–9.

50. Cronin J, McNair PJ, Marshall RN. Velocity specificity, combination training and sport specific tasks. J Sci Med Sport 2001;4(2):168–78.

51. Bell GJ, Petersen SR, Quinney HA, et al. The effect of velocity-specific strength training on peak torque and anaerobic rowing power. J Sports Sci 1989;7(3):205–14.

52. Young WB, Rath DA. Enhancing foot velocity in football kicking: the role of strength training. J Strength Cond Res 2011;25(2):561–6.

53. Behm DG, Sale DG. Velocity specificity of resistance training. Sports Med 1993;15(6):374–88.

54. Farlinger CM, Fowles JR. The effect of sequence of skating-specific training on skating performance. Int J Sports Physiol Perform 2008;3(2):185–98.

55. Bloomfield J, Blanksby BA, Ackland TR, et al.. The influence of strength training on overhead throwing velocity of elite water polo players. Aust J Sci Med Sport 1990;22(3):63–7.

56. Wilson GJ, Murphy AJ, Walshe A. The specificity of strength training: the effect of posture. Eur J Appl Physiol Occup Physiol 1996;73(3–4):346–52.

57. Asseman F, Caron O, Cremieux J. Is there a transfer of postural ability from specific to unspecific postures in elite gymnasts? Neurosci Lett 2004;358:83–6.

58. Paillard T, Costes-Salon MC, Lafont C, et al. Are there differences in postural regulation according to the level of competition in judoists? Br J Sports Med 2002;36:304–5.

59. Paillard T, Noe F, Riviere T. Performance and strategy in the unipedal stance of soccer players at different levels of competition. J Athl Train 2006;41(2):172–6.

60. Simmons RW. Sensory organization determinants of postural stability in trained ballet dancers. Int J Neurosci 2005;115(1):87–97.
61. Flynn MG, Pizza FX, Boone JB Jr, et al. Indices of training stress during competitive running and swimming seasons. Int J Sports Med 1994;15(1):21–6.
62. Pizza FX, Flynn MG, Starling RD, et al. Run training vs cross training: influence of increased training on running economy, foot impact shock and run performance. Int J Sports Med 1995;16(3):180–4.
63. Mutton DL, Loy SF, Rogers DM, et al. Effect of run vs combined cycle/run training on VO2max and running performance. Med Sci Sports Exerc 1993;25(12):1393–7.
64. Godges JJ, MacRae PG, Engelke KA. Effects of exercise on hip range of motion, trunk muscle performance, and gait economy. Phys Ther 1993;73(7):468–77.
65. King JA, Cipriani DJ. Comparing preseason frontal and sagittal plane plyometric programs on vertical jump height in high-school basketball players. J Strength Cond Res 2010;24(8):2109–14.
66. Krzystzof N, Waskiewicz Z, Zajac A, et al. The effects of exhaustive bench press on bimanual coordination. In: Lee CP, editor. Proceedings of 2nd international conference on weightlifting and strength training; 2000:86.
67. Magnusson P, Renstro P. The European College of Sports Sciences position statement: the role of stretching exercises in sports. Eur J Sport Sci 2006;6(2):87–91.
68. Ingraham SJ. The role of flexibility in injury prevention and athletic performance: have we stretched the truth? Minn Med 2003;86(5):58–61.
69. Kay AD, Blazevich AJ. Effect of acute static stretch on maximal muscle performance: a systematic review. Med Sci Sports Exerc 2012;44(1):154–64.
70. Higgs F, Winter SL. The effect of a four-week proprioceptive neuromuscular facilitation stretching program on isokinetic torque production. J Strength Cond Res 2009;23(5):1442–7.
71. Hunter JP, Marshall RN. Effects of power and flexibility training on within-task–task jump technique. Med Sci Sports Exerc 2002;34(3):478–86.
72. Yuktasir B, Kaya F. Investigation into the long-term effects of static and PNF stretching exercises on range of motion and jump performance. J Bodyw Mov Ther 2009;13:11–21.
73. Wilson GJ, Elliott BC, Wood GA. Stretch shorten cycle performance enhancement through flexibility training. Med Sci Sports Exerc 1992;24(1):116–23.
74. Falla D, Jull G, Hodges P. Training the cervical muscles with prescribed motor tasks does not change muscle activation during a functional activity. Man Ther 2008;13(6):507–12.
75. Rotem-Lehrer N, Laufer Y. Effect of focus of attention on transfer of a postural control task following an ankle sprain. J Orthop Sports Phys Ther 2007;37(9):564–9.
76. Sullivan KJ, Brown DA, Klassen T, et al. Effects of task-specific locomotor and strength training in adults who were ambulatory after stroke: results of the STEPS randomized clinical trial. Phys Ther 2007;87(12):1580–602, 1603–7.
77. Flansbjer UB, Miller M, Downham D, et al. Progressive resistance training after stroke: effects on muscle strength, muscle tone, gait performance and perceived participation. J Rehabil Med 2008;40(1):42–8.
78. Dean CM, Channon EF, Hall JM. Sitting training early after stroke improves sitting ability and quality and carries over to standing up but not to walking: a randomised trial. Aust J Physiother 2007;53(2):97–102.
79. van de Port IG, Wood-Dauphinee S, Lindeman E, et al. Effects of exercise training programs on walking competency after stroke: a systematic review. Am J Phys Med Rehabil 2007;86(11):935–51.
80. Van Peppen RP, Kwakkel G, Wood-Dauphinee S, et al. The impact of physical therapy on functional outcomes after stroke: what's the evidence? Clin Rehabil 2004;18(8):833–62.
81. Bogey R, Hornby GT. Gait training strategies utilized in poststroke rehabilitation: are we really making a difference? Top Stroke Rehabil 2007;14(6):1–8.

82. de Haart M, Geurts AC, Huidekoper SC, et al. Recovery of standing balance in postacute stroke patients: a rehabilitation cohort study. Arch Phys Med Rehabil 2004;85(6): 886–95.

83. Sherrington C, Whitney JC, Lord SR, et al. Effective exercise for the prevention of falls: a systematic review and meta-analysis. J Am Geriatr Soc 2008;56:2234–43.

84. Genthon N, Rougier P, Gissot AS, et al. Contribution of each lower limb to upright standing in stroke patients. Stroke 2008;39(6):1793–9.

85. Reis JG, Costa GC, Schmidt A, et al. Do muscle strengthening exercises improve performance in the 6-minute walk test in postmenopausal women? Rev Bras Fisioter 2012;16(3):236–40.

86. Christiansen CL. The effects of hip and ankle stretching on gait function of older people. Arch Phys Med Rehabil 2008;89:1421–8.

87. Hartmann A, Murer K, de Bie RA, et al. The effect of a foot gymnastic exercise programme on gait performance in older adults: a randomised controlled trial. Disabil Rehabil 2009;31(25):2101–10.

88. Watt JR, Jackson K, Franz JR, et al. Effect of a supervised hip flexor stretching program on gait in frail elderly patients. PM R 2011;3(4):330–5.

89. Kerrigan DC, Lee LW, Collins JJ, et al. Reduced hip extension during walking: healthy elderly and fallers versus young adults. Arch Phys Med Rehabil 2001;82:26–30.

90. Kerrigan DC, Todd MK, Della Croce U, et al. Biomechanical gait alterations independent of speed in the healthy elderly: evidence for specific limiting impairments. Arch Phys Med Rehabil 1998;79:317–22.

91. Katalinic OM, Harvey LA, Herbert RD. Effectiveness of stretch for the treatment and prevention of contractures in people with neurological conditions: a systematic review. Phys Ther 2011;91(1):11–24.

92. Hubbard IJ, Parsons MW, Neilson C, et al. Task-specific training: evidence for and translation to clinical practice. Occup Ther Int 2009;16(3–4):175–89.

93. Muehlbauer T, Panzer S, Shea CH. The transfer of movement sequences: effects of decreased and increased load. Q J Exp Psychol 2007;60(6):770–8.

94. Dean NJ, Kovacs AJ, Shea CH. Transfer of movement sequences: bigger is better. Acta Psychol 2008;127(2):355–68.

95. Buchanan JJ, Zihlman K, Ryu YU, et al. Learning and transfer of a relative phase pattern and a joint amplitude ratio in a rhythmic multijoint arm movement. J Mot Behav 2007;39(1):49–67.

96. Leirdal S, Roeleveld K, Ettema G. Coordination specificity in strength and power training. Int J Sports Med 2008;29(3):225–31.

97. Chandler JM, Duncan PW, Kochersberger G, et al. Is lower extremity strength gain associated with improvement in physical performance and disability in frail, community-dwelling elders? Arch Phys Med Rehabil 1998;79(1):24–30.

98. Host HH, Sinacore DR, Bohnert KL, et al. Strength and function improved with exercise after hip fracture. Phys Ther 2007;87(3):292–303.

99. Kalapotharakos VI, Topmakidis SP, Smilios I, et al. Resistance training in older women: effect on within-task–task jump and functional performance. J Sports Med Phys Fitness 2005;45(4):570–5.

100. Kalapotharakos VI, Michalopoulos M, Tokmakidis SP, et al. Effects of a heavy and a moderate resistance training on functional performance in older adults. J Strength Cond Res 2005;19(3):652–7.

101. Liu CJ, Latham NK. Progressive resistance strength training for improving physical function in older adults. Cochrane Database Syst Rev 2009;3:CD002759.

102. Loy SF, Hoffmann JJ, Holland GJ. Benefits and practical use of cross-training in sports. Sports Med 1995;19(1):1–8.

103. Manini T, Marko M, VanArnam T, et al. Efficacy of resistance and task-specific exercise in older adults who modify tasks of everyday life. J Gerontol A Biol Sci Med Sci 2007;62(6): 616–23.

104. de Vreede PL, Samson MM, van Meeteren NL, et al. Functional-task exercise versus resistance strength exercise to improve daily function in older women: a randomized, controlled trial. J Am Geriatr Soc 2005;53(1):2–10.
105. Bean JF, Herman S, Kiely DK, et al. Increased velocity exercise specific to task (InVEST) training: a pilot study exploring effects on leg power, balance, and mobility in community-dwelling older women. J Am Geriatr Soc 2004;52(5):799–804.
106. Bean JF, Kiely DK, LaRose S, et al. Increased velocity exercise specific to task training versus the National Institute on Aging's strength training program: changes in limb power and mobility. J Gerontol A Biol Sci Med Sci 2009;64(9):983–91.
107. Skelton DA, Young A, Greig CA, et al. Effects of resistance training on strength, power, and selected functional abilities of women aged 75 and older. J Am Geriatr Soc 1995;43(10): 1081–7.
108. Blennerhassett J, Dite W. Additional task-related practice improves mobility and upper limb function early after stroke: a randomised controlled trial. Aust J Physiother 2004;50: 219–24.
109. Shea CH, Kohl RM. Specificity and variability of practice. Res Q Exerc Sport 1990;61(2): 169–77.
110. Livesey JP, Laszlo JI. Effect of task similarity on transfer performance. J Mot Behav 1979;11(1):11–21.
111. Hall KG, Magill RA. Variability of practice and contextual interference in motor skill learning. J Mot Behav 1995;27(4):299–309.
112. Porter JM, Magill RA. Systematically increasing contextual interference is beneficial for learning sport skills. J Sports Sci 2010;14:1–9.
113. Green DP, Whitehead J, Sugden DA. Practice variability and transfer of a racket skill. Percept Mot Skills 1995;81(3 Pt 2):1275–81.
114. Brady F. Contextual interference: a meta-analytic study. Percept Mot Skills 2004;99(1): 116–26.
115. Maslovat M, Chua R, Lee TD, et al. Contextual interference: single task versus multi-task learning. Motor Control 2004;8:213–33.
116. Dick MB, Hsieh S, Dick-Muehlke C. The variability of practice hypothesis in motor learning: does it apply to Alzheimer's disease? Brain Cogn 2000;44(3):470–89.
117. Dick MB, Hsieh S, Bricker J. Facilitating acquisition and transfer of a continuous motor task in healthy older adults and patients with Alzheimer's disease. Neuropsychology 2003;17(2):202–12.
118. Lin CH, Sullivan KJ, Wu AD, et al. Effect of task practice order on motor skill learning in adults with Parkinson disease: a pilot study. Phys Ther 2007;87(9):1120–31.
119. Totsika V, Wulf G. The influence of external and internal foci of attention on transfer to novel situations and skills. Res Q Exerc Sport 2003;74(2):220–5.
120. McEwen SE, Polatajko HJ, Huijbregts MP, et al. Inter-task transfer of meaningful, functional skills following a cognitive-based treatment: results of three multiple baseline design experiments in adults with chronic stroke. Neuropsychol Rehabil 2010;20(4):541–61.
121. Shadmehr R, Maurice A, Smith MA, et al. Error correction, sensory prediction, and adaptation in motor control. Annu Rev Neurosci 2010;33:89–108.
122. Yoshida M, Cauraugh JH, Chow JW. Specificity of practice, visual information, and intersegmental dynamics in rapid-aiming limb movements. J Mot Behav 2004;36(3):281–90.
123. Khan MA, Franks IM, Goodman D. The effect of practice on the control of rapid aiming movements: evidence for an interdependency between programming and feedback processing. Q J Exp Psychol Hum Exp Psychol 1998;51A:425–44.
124. Klam F, Graf W. Vestibular signals of posterior parietal cortex neurons during active and passive head movements in macaque monkeys. Ann NY Acad Sci 2003;1004:271–82.
125. Elliott D, Grierson LE, Hayes SJ, et al. Action representations in perception, motor control and learning: implications for medical education. Med Educ 2011;45(2):119–31.
126. Elliott D, Hansen S, Grierson LE, et al. Goal-directed aiming: two components but multiple processes. Psychol Bull 2010;136(6):1023–44.

127. Asseman FB, Caron O, Crémieux J. Are there specific conditions for which expertise in gymnastics could have an effect on postural control and performance? Gait Posture 2008;27(1): 76–81.

128. Robertson S, Elliott D. Specificity of learning and dynamic balance. Res Q Exerc Sport 1996;67(1):69–75.

129. Carey LM, Matyas TA, Oke LE. Sensory loss in stroke patients: effective tactile and proprioceptive discrimination training. Arch Phys Med Rehabil 1993;74:602–11.

130. Carey LM, Matyas TA. Training of somatosensory discrimination after stroke: facilitation of stimulus generalization. Am J Phys Med Rehabil 2005;84(6):428–42.

131. Carey LM, Matyas TA. Frequency of discriminative sensory loss in the hand after stroke in a rehabilitation setting. J Rehabil Med 2011;43(3):257–63.

132. Tremblay L, Proteau L. Specificity of practice in a ball interception task. Can J Exp Psychol 2001;55(3):207–18.

133. Mackrous I, Proteau L. Specificity of practice results from differences in movement planning strategies. Exp Brain Res 2007;183(2):181–93.

134. Robin C, Toussaint L, Blandin Y, et al. Specificity of learning in a video-aiming task: modifying the salience of dynamic visual cues. J Mot Behav 2005;37(5):367–76.

135. Proteau L, Tremblay L, Dejaeger D. Practice does not diminish the role of visual information in on-line control of a precision walking task: support for the specificity of practice hypothesis. J Mot Behav 2005;30(2):143–50.

136. Sathian K, Zangaladze A. Tactile learning is task specific but transfers between fingers. Percept Psychophys 1997;59:119–28.

137. Grant AC, Thiagarajah MC, Sathian K. Tactile perception in blind Braille readers: a psychophysical study of acuity and hyperacuity using gratings and dot patterns. Percept Psychophys 2000;62(2):301–12.

138. Carel C, Loubinoux I, Boulanouar K, et al. Neural substrate for the effects of passive training on sensorimotor cortical representation: a study with functional magnetic resonance imaging in healthy subjects. J Cereb Blood Flow Metab 2000;20(3):478–84.

139. Macé MJ, Levin O, Alaerts K, et al. Corticospinal facilitation following prolonged proprioceptive stimulation by means of passive wrist movement. J Clin Neurophysiol 2008;25(4): 202–9.

140. Lewis GN, Byblow WD. The effects of repetitive proprioceptive stimulation on corticomotor representation in intact and hemiplegic individuals. Clin Neurophysiol 2004;115(4):765–73.

141. Cambier DC, De Corte E, Danneels LA, et al. Treating sensory impairments in the post-stroke upper limb with intermittent pneumatic compression: results of a preliminary trial. Clin Rehabil 2003;17(1):14–20.

142. Doyle S, Bennett S, Fasoli SE, et al. Interventions for sensory impairment in the upper limb after stroke. Cochrane Database Syst Rev 2010;6:CD006331.

CHAPTER 6

The Overloading Condition for Recovery

To write this book I have spent many hours sitting over several years, in mostly flexed slouched position. Yet, the flexion range of my back has remained unchanged. Nor do prolonged weight-bearing activities such as standing result in permanent flattening of the medial arches of my feet. In these and many other postural activities, prolonged high levels of stresses are imposed on the body, yet range of movement (ROM) does not seem to increase. If such levels of postural stress do not bring about a permanent range change why should we expect it to occur by manual stretching or exercise? Yet, paradoxically, yoga practitioners and ballet dancers seem to overcome this physiological barrier to gain remarkable flexibility. Is there something we can learn from them?

This chapter will explore the overloading condition for tissue adaptation, including:

- What force levels drive tissue adaptation?
- How much force is required to maintain the functional ROM?
- How much force is required during ROM rehabilitation?
- What are the safe levels of force during stretching? Can they be assessed?
- Can manual therapy techniques provide sufficient forces for long-term flexibility?

LOADING LEVELS AND THRESHOLDS

Long ago, I trained in martial arts and later as a yoga teacher – two disciplines that required a high level of flexibility. The magnitude of force seems to have played an important role in this training. A full forward bending was achieved by pulling forcefully on my feet while the instructor sat on my back. That seemed to have worked well. From just being able to touch my knees, I was able to bend my back and flatten my chest against my outstretched legs, amongst other great feats of agility. These gains in flexibility took several months to attain and several years to perfect. This personal experience suggests that, *for effective long-term tissue elongation, the force of*

73

ROM challenges must be above the forces imposed by normal functional demands. Otherwise, we would gradually be turned into dysfunctional hyperflexible masses by the daily stresses imposed on our bodies. This experience also suggests that force interacts with the duration and frequency of stretching. This will be discussed in Chapter 7.

From the example above we can start exploring the forces that are required for tissue adaptation (Fig. 6.1). The first premise is that the functional ROM is maintained by the forces imposed on the body by daily activities, termed here *functional loading forces*. In order to increase performance/conditioning beyond the daily defaults, the intensity of the activity has to increase – *overloading*. For example, in the Achilles tendon, adaptation is only observed when loading forces exceed the normal daily values.[1] Forces below the functional level, *underloading*, result in atrophy and loss of ROM.[2] Between the functional and overloading levels is an *overloading threshold*. Between the functional and underloading levels is a *functional threshold*. So daily activity maintains functional ROM. To increase ROM the forces have to reach some overloading threshold, whereas reducing physical activities below the functional threshold will result in deconditioning.

The question that arises is how do we assess loading levels? Where is the threshold? Is there a way to identify it? Unfortunately, such an assessment is clinically improbable. The main feedback or guidance for loading is ultimately discomfort. As discussed in Chapter 2, functional activities are mostly performed within a comfortable movement range (comfort zone) (Fig. 6.1), whereas overloading is often associated with some level of discomfort. It is

Overloading	ROM increase	Discomfort zone
Overloading threshold		
Functional loading	Functional ROM	Comfort zone
Functional loading threshold		
Underloading	ROM loss/atrophy	

FIGURE 6.1 Functional loading, overloading and underloading. Functional loading imposed during daily activities provides sufficient stimulation to maintain the functional range of movement (ROM). These stresses are often within a comfort zone of movement. To increase ROM beyond the functional ranges, overloading is required. These challenges are often within a discomfort zone. Underloading below a functional level often results in atrophy and loss of ROM.

often our main feedback during exercise but also during ROM challenges: we assume that patient discomfort represents the point at which overloading takes place. As will be discussed later in this chapter and in Chapter 9, discomfort is an imperfect and inaccurate guide, but there is little else we can use to estimate loading levels.

Overloading in relation to ROM loss and recovery

It is well established that in frozen shoulder the patient will recover their ROM over time and without assistance.[3] This means that range improvement is possible by performing functional tasks, but where is the overloading threshold in this recovery?

There is the possibility that lower loading thresholds are required when ROM losses are present. In contractures, the restricted end-range may represent a lowered functional threshold. This means that normal daily activities that require greater ROM may provide the forces and ranges necessary to challenge this threshold (Fig. 6.2). For example, in the ankle during walking, the normal total dorsiflexion and plantarflexion range is about 30°.[4] If, because of contractures, this range drops to, say, 20°, this would represent a lowered functional threshold. In this situation, walking, which requires 30°, may generate sufficient loading forces to challenge the limited range. Walking on a steep, sloped surface and stairs could further raise the functional loading levels.[4,5]

In the presence of ROM losses there is often a shift in the discomfort zone to include the functional range of activities (Fig. 6.2). In the example above, the ROM losses in the ankle are likely to be accompanied by discomfort during functional activities such as walking or climbing stairs. The patient should be made aware that this is normal and even desirable.

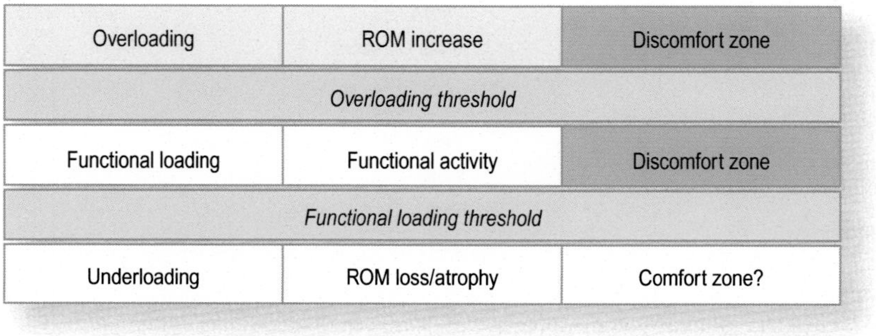

Overloading	ROM increase	Discomfort zone
Overloading threshold		
Functional loading	Functional activity	Discomfort zone
Functional loading threshold		
Underloading	ROM loss/atrophy	Comfort zone?

FIGURE 6.2 Functional loading may provide sufficient challenge in the presence of adaptive range of movement (ROM) losses. Under these circumstances the functional challenge will be within the discomfort zone.

Impediments to overloading

Sensitivity/pain and failure to provide sufficient force are common factors that may interfere with overloading during ROM rehabilitation.

ROM losses are often accompanied by pain and anxieties about movement (Chs 9 and 10). Under these circumstances, the patient may terminate the stretching well before it reaches the necessary loading thresholds. This can be resolved partly by dissociating the discomfort from the damage and by focusing on alleviating pain levels before commencing the ROM challenge programme (Ch. 9). For example, in frozen shoulder, the ROM challenges can start when the condition is no longer in the painful phase.

Another impediment is related to the failure of many traditional stretching approaches to generate sufficient forces to reach the loading thresholds (Table 6.1). For example, techniques such as side-lying flexion articulation or manipulation of the spine are unlikely to result in any permanent increase in range (except for the inconsequential elongation discussed below). Such manually applied forces are nowhere close to those imposed by bending and lifting or sitting. The capsular ligaments of the apophyseal joints can by themselves support twice the body weight.[6] Failure to generate sufficient forces can be encountered elsewhere in the body. The Achilles tendon or the plantar fascia can withstand considerable forces during functional activities. In walking, the vertical forces on the foot are 1–1.5 times the body weight, in running 2–3

Table 6.1 Potential of different range of movement (ROM) challenges to provide sufficient loading for adaptation. With some of the passive approaches it may be possible but it depends on the therapist's ability to generate enough force and the area of the body being stretched

	Management/ROM challenge	Does it provide sufficient loading?	
Functional	Recovery behaviour	**Yes**	Most effective
	Managed recovery behaviour	**Yes**	
	Assisted recovery behaviour (functional stretching)	**Yes**	
Extra-functional	Ballistic stretching	**Yes**	
	Dynamic stretching	**Yes**	
	Muscle energy techniques	**Yes**	
	Passive stretching	No	
	Spinal manipulation	No	
	Traction	No	
	Articulation	No	
	Harmonic	No	
	Strain counter-strain	No	
	Cranial	No	Least effective

times the body weight and during a triple jump 7–12 times the body weight.[7,8] A therapist is likely to injure their hands long before the functional thresholds are reached during stretching. In patients with adaptive ROM losses, the practical solution is to exploit daily activities and to amplify them to provide the necessary loading forces (Ch. 12).

On the lower spectrum of loading inefficacy are manual therapy approaches that use minimal force to promote long-term tissue changes. They include techniques such as strain counter-strain and craniosacral and facial unwinding techniques. In cranial approaches, it is believed that the position and movement of the cranial bones can be modified by gentle manual handling/holding of the head. If such forces were effective then wearing a hat or resting the head on a pillow would result in serious distortions of the skull – if it does not happen by (recurrent) functional stresses, it will not happen by weaker (occasional) manual forces.

The "inconsequential" elongation

Try this home experiment: stretch your index finger into full extension and maintain that angle. After a short while you will experience a certain "give" in resistance. When this happens the joint can be stretched further without any additional force (creep deformation; Fig. 6.3A) or maintained at the same position with less force (force relaxation; Fig 6.3B).[9–15] This drop in resistance is related to a biomechanical property of muscle and connective tissues called

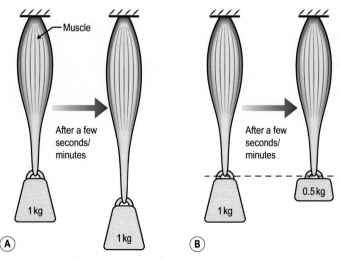

FIGURE 6.3 A. Creep deformation. B. Force relaxation. Both are related to the viscoelastic properties of tissues.

viscoelasticity.[16-18] Musculoskeletal tissues are composed of fibres embedded within a viscous, gel-like medium.[14,15,19-22] The fibrous elements provide strength and resistance during loading. The viscous gel elements endow the tissues with a slow, flow-like elongation experienced during stretching (Box 6.1).[23]

Creep deformation and force relaxation can be observed during all forms of tensional loading.[24,25] During sustained muscle stretching creep deformation accounts for 75–85% of the elongation that occurs within the first 15–20 seconds.[23] In cyclical stretching about 80% of the elongation will take place in the first four repetitions.[19,26] This is often experienced during stretching exercise; most of the range gains occur within the first three or four repetitions, after which the range gains tend to plateau. Force relaxation has been demonstrated in the anterior longitudinal ligament of the spine and during sustained dorsiflexion of the ankle. The force needed to maintain the longitudinal ligament at a given tension halved within the first minute of loading.[16] In the ankle joint it takes about 5 minutes to achieve full force relaxation.[27]

The viscoelastic behaviour of tissues can be deceptive to the therapist and patient. It gives the impression that stretching culminates in longer fibres. However, the immediate change in ROM during stretching is not due to true length changes in the tissue. All that happens is that the tissue has transformed from a stiff into a "softer", more compliant spring, which means that for a given force it can extend further (Fig. 6.4). These viscoelastic changes in the tissue are transient. At the termination of stretching the tissues will gradually return to their original biomechanical/structural state (Fig. 6.4). The rate at which this recovery occurs varies between tissues. In the hamstrings force relaxation recovers within an hour, whereas in the Achilles tendon it will take several hours.[9-11,27-29]

These viscoelastic responses are biomechanical events. They are not associated with adaptive elongation, a process that occurs in the biological dimension (Ch. 5). Such viscoelastic length changes are therefore "inconsequential" for long-term ROM recovery. The inconsequential elongation is expected to be present immediately after any kind of manual stretching techniques, joint manipulation or exercise.[30] However, range increases that are present for longer than a few hours after the session are more likely to be associated with other physiological mechanisms, such as an increased tolerance to the sensation of stretching (Ch. 10), or contextual effects/placebos (Ch. 9).

The inconsequential elongation creates a paradox: how can long-term elongation take place if tissues return to their original length shortly after the cessation of loading? Long-term ROM adaptation occurs when this mechanical signal is repeated by successive episodes of tension loading (mechanotransduction, Ch 4). So, by itself, a single overloading episode will be insufficient.

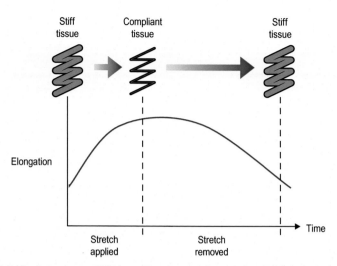

FIGURE 6.4 The inconsequential elongation. In acute bouts of stretching the immediate elongation is associated with a creep response, a transient biomechanical event associated with viscoelasticity. The elongation is due to a change in stiffness rather than a true length change in the tissues.

The duration and repetition element of the ROM challenge will be discussed in Chapter 7.

Rate of stretching

The rate of stretching is another consideration that often troubles physical therapists. Should it be slow, as in yoga, or rapid, as in ballistic stretching?

The level of resistance in the tissue can change in response to different velocities of stretching.[16,18,19] During slow stretching the tissue undergoes a viscous, flow-like length change. At higher velocities of stretching the tissue behaves more like a stiff spring, with increasing velocities resulting in greater resistance (Fig. 6.5).[31] Furthermore, less force is required to achieve greater length during slow stretching.[32] In animal tendons, a low-load sustained stretching is more effective at producing elongation than a high-load brief stretch.[33] In flexion contractures in the knee, low-load sustained stretching was shown to be more effective than brief high-load stretching in producing short-term elongation.[34]

So which is better, spinal manipulation or a slow sustained stretch? Spinal manipulation is a high-velocity stretch, so from a biomechanical perspective a sustained stretch may be more effective. However, all this may be trivial. These velocity-dependent tissue responses are a transient biomechanical phenomenon associated with the inconsequential elongation rather than tissue adaptation.

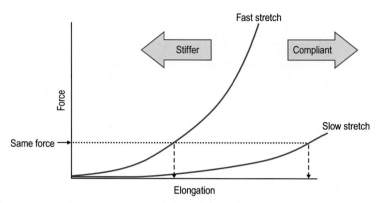

FIGURE 6.5 The rate of loading will influence the resistance experienced during stretching. At a given force, slower stretching will result in greater elongation than higher stretching velocities.

Where rate of loading may be important is in relation to specificity of training and the goal task. Slow stretching to the end-range may be suitable for yoga but not for fast kicking in martial arts. This is related to the specificity phenomenon in training and motor learning discussed in Chapter 5.

The "undesirable" plastic ROM change

There is an enduring belief in manual therapy that tissue damage is essential for long-term length changes. It is hypothesized that stretching causes connective tissue or muscle damage. This in turn would initiate a repair process that, when combined with end-range challenges, would culminate in tissue elongation.[35]

Damage to connective tissue is expected to occur somewhere in the elastic and in the plastic range, depending on the tissue stretched (Box 6.2). At this point, some of the fibres will begin to tear. When stretching is removed the tissue will not return to its original length and would be more compliant, owing to a lower number of intact fibres. This would indeed result in a range increase but at the cost of tissue damage and inflammation. Whether such tissue destructive approaches are necessary is doubtful. It is known that ROM losses can often recover by normal functional use without evidence of damage–repair cycles.[36] Such biomechanical adaptation in muscle and connective tissue can occur by mechanotransduction, which is not associated with tissue damage. (Ch. 4). Hence, imposing damage as a therapeutic approach is not clinically justifiable.

Another common belief is that stretching can be used to tear adhesions and overcome contractures. However, within a few weeks, adhesions can have greater strength than the tissues to which they are attached. Similarly, contractures undergo biomechanical changes that result in less extensible tissue.

Table 6.2 Mechanisms underlying range of movement (ROM) improvements. The biological adaptive process should be the target of ROM rehabilitation

		Duration	Tissue damage?	Permanent?
Biomechanical	Creep deformation	Few seconds to minutes	No	No
	Plastic	Few seconds to minutes	Temporary (recovery by repair but may leave permanent damage)	Yes
Biological	Adaptation	Weeks, months	No	Yes

Hence, imposing an acute bout of stretching to break adhesions may cause damage to surrounding healthy tissues. In contractures, it will result in converting a stiff, but often intact, structure into a damaged one. For example, manipulation under anaesthesia for frozen shoulder results in extensive damage to multiple joint structures.[37] In a group of 30 patients it was found that after manipulation 11 had superior capsule ruptures, 24 had anterior capsule ruptures up to the infraglenoid pole, 16 had posterior capsular lesions, four had superior labrum tears, three had partial tears of the subscapularis tendon, four had anterior labral detachments and two patients had tears of the middle glenohumeral ligament. So damage does immediately increase the joint ROM but at a frightening cost to joint integrity.

The mechanisms underlying ROM improvements are summarized in Table 6.2.

GRADED CHALLENGE AND THE TASK PARAMETERS

After an injury most individuals will return to pre-injury activities in a gradual manner. They take a series of graded challenges that are amplified over time. Positive movement experiences embolden them to increase the level of challenge. For example, a person with a shoulder injury will incrementally increase the *force*, *range* and *velocity* of lifting. As they improve they will also tend to increase the repetition of lifting. This represents the *endurance* parameter that is necessary to maintain or repeat the task.

This positive recovery behaviour can be applied clinically in the form of a graded ROM challenge (Fig. 6.6). In this approach these four movement parameters (force, range, velocity and endurance) are overloaded or amplified in an incremental manner (Fig. 6.7). For example, for the frozen shoulder patient the physical challenge can be to hold a bottle of water with the affected side and repetitively reach and place it on the therapist's hands, as if reaching to place it on a shelf (Ch. 13). During the reaching movement, the therapist changes the positions of the hands to challenge the four task parameters. The

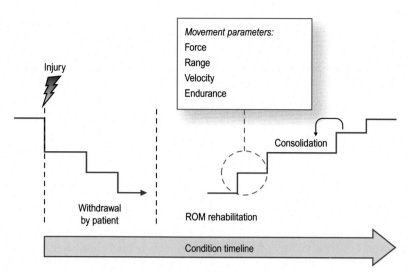

FIGURE 6.6 Graded overloading and amplification of the four task parameters: force, range, velocity and endurance. ROM, range of movement.

Date:
Name:

	Week 1	Week 2	Week 3	Week 4	Week 5	Week 6	Week 7	Week 8	Week 9
Tennis	Distance from wall: **3m** Duration: **5 min** Frequency: **× 3**	Distance from wall: **4m** Duration: **5 min** Frequency: **× 3**	Distance from wall: **5m** Duration: **5 min** Frequency: **× 3**	Distance from wall: **5m** Duration: **10 min** Frequency: **× 3**	Distance from wall: **5m** Duration: **15 min** Frequency: **× 3**	Distance from wall: **5m** Duration: **20 min** Frequency: **× 3**	Distance from wall: **Any distance** Duration: **25 min** Frequency: **× 3**	Start a 5–10 minute game with a partner, just passing the ball	Etc.

Amplifying force — spanning Weeks 1–3 / *Amplifying endurance* — spanning Weeks 4–8

FIGURE 6.7 Graded challenge in clinic using tennis as an example. Here, force and endurance are amplified within the task.

Date:
Name:

	Week 1	Week 2	Week 3	Week 4	Week 5	Week 6	Week 7	Week 8	Week 9	Week 10	Week 11	Week 12
Tennis	Start here											
Swimming				Start here								
Cycling								Start here				

FIGURE 6.8 Graded challenge for several activities using staggering. Patients dictate exercise priorities.

range parameter can be challenged by the therapist moving their hands further away from the patient to a position above their head (extension–flexion) and to their side (abduction–adduction). Velocity can be challenged by performing the reaching movements faster; endurance by increasing the number of repetitions; and force by using progressively heavier objects. Later, other activities can be added in a staggered manner (Fig. 6.8). So, the principle of overloading is extended to include amplification of the four movement parameters but also incrementally adding activities; overloading is not just about force.

The graded challenge provides a consolidation time for adaptation to take place and reduces the potential for re-injury.[38,39] This is achieved by the incremental overloading/amplification of the four movement parameters within comfortable/tolerable ranges. When an adverse reaction is encountered, the graded challenge can be dropped back a step (Fig. 6.6). During the consolidation period, the patient maintains the activity at that level. After, say, 2 or 3 weeks they are then encouraged to move up a step. An adverse reaction can be set as being greater than 2–3 points on a 0–10 pain scale and lasting more than, for example, a day or two. Incremental ROM is particularly important in situations where there is a history of recent tissue damage, such as after surgery. A graded challenge has an important role in reassuring the patient as well as the therapist that the movement is safe, and in providing positive movement experiences that contribute to the narrative of success (Ch. 11).

THE FALLACY OF SPECIFIC TISSUE STRETCHING/LOADING

Specific tissue stretching is often promoted as a valued clinical skill in physical therapy education. There is an enduring belief that individual muscles, fascias or joint capsules can be stretched/loaded to the exclusion of others. However, is such specificity therapeutically desirable and is it physically possible?

There is no obvious clinical rationale for specific tissue stretching. In contractures, all tissues undergo adaptive changes. Hence, it is far more beneficial to load simultaneously all the affected tissues.

It is doubtful whether stretching specificity is possible. It is a misconception largely derived from anatomy and physical therapy education. Anatomy books tend to illustrate structures that are well defined and separated from their surrounding tissues. This gives rise to the false impression that muscles, tendons and fascias are detached from each other and separated by anatomical voids. In reality, tissues and structures are extensively connected and closely compacted. When a force, such as stretching, is applied all the tissues are loaded simultaneously. Even if single muscle stretching were possible, it is expected that the tensional forces will be transmitted via the extensive fascial connections to adjacent and even antagonistic muscle groups.[40–42]

Specific tissue loading is improbable and clinically irrational. The focus of ROM rehabilitation should be on the movement affected rather than the tissues/muscles that impede this range. For example, in glenohumeral contracture the focus should be on recovering overhead arm movements rather than attempting to stretch each individual tissue that contributes to this restriction. Functional overhead challenges have the advantage of loading all the affected tissues simultaneously. This approach reduces clinical complexity and the need for muscle-by-muscle rehabilitation.

SUMMARY

- Functional ROM is maintained by the forces imposed on the body by daily activities
- Overloading is a training condition for adaptation in which physical challenges are raised above functional levels
- Forces below the overload threshold will be ineffective at inducing long-term ROM change
- Underloading is the absence of sufficient forces required to maintain functional activities; it results in atrophy and adaptive ROM loss
- Functional activities may generate sufficient forces in conditions where adaptive ROM losses are present
- Many manual stretching approaches may fail to generate sufficient force for overloading; active, functional activities should be used whenever possible
- Functional activities and managed recovery behaviour may provide sufficient forces for adaptive ROM recovery
- The four movement parameters (force, range, speed and endurance) are the target of overloading and amplification
- Amplification and overloading should be introduced in a graded manner – a graded challenge
- Overloading is associated with the experience of discomfort

- Functional and overloading thresholds cannot be assessed clinically; discomfort is the principal feedback for loading
- Overloading is likely to be unpleasant. Patients who are in pain or who have movement-related fears may not tolerate stretching and may terminate it before the loading threshold is reached; pain alleviation may be necessary before vigorous ROM challenges commence
- Just because it feels like a stretch does not mean that it is effective
- Message to the patient – "just keep on moving, discomfort is OK, it will help it get better"

BOX 6.1 STRETCHING TERMS EXPLAINED

There are several terms that are often used to describe what happens during stretching which can be confusing and often get mixed up. They include tensile strength, stiff, compliant, elastic, flexible and force and strength.

Generally, the term *tensile strength* describes how much force a tissue can withstand before it fails. The term *strength* can often be mixed up with muscle strength, which is the force generated by muscle contraction. This mix-up can lead to misconceptions such as that spinal strength can be improved by exercise which increases trunk muscle strength. The spinal discs and ligaments have inherent tensile strength, which is not directly related to the person's ability to lift a heavy weight.

Stiff and *compliant* are terms used to describe the resistance of a tissue or joint during bending/stretching. Imagine stretching two different tissues using the same force (Fig. 6.9). One tissue will elongate more than the other. The tissue which elongates most is said to be compliant in comparison with the one which elongated least – the stiffer tissue. However, this compliance does not necessarily relate to their tensile strength. A tissue can be highly compliant yet have higher tensile strength than a tissue that feels stiffer when stretched (Fig. 6.10).

There is another potential mix-up with the term *stiffness*. There is biomechanical and subjective stiffness. Biomechanical stiffness is the physical resistance of the tissue to an applied load. Subjective stiffness is the sense of effort or the level of discomfort that a person experiences when stretching or bending. It can be partly related to the underlying biomechanical stiffness; however, in many conditions a subjective sense of stiffness is due to increased sensitivity of the tissues under tension from injury or localized swelling, rather than shortening of the tissues. So although the tissue feels stiffer it might be damaged and weaker (Ch. 9). In this situation stretching should be avoided since nothing is stiffer or shorter; it just feels like that.

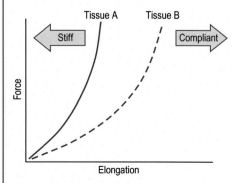

FIGURE 6.9 Stiffness and compliance.

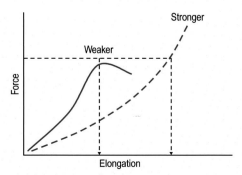

FIGURE 6.10 Tensile strength.

BOX 6.2   BIOMECHANICS OF STRETCHING

Physical forces can be applied to the body in the form of tension and/or compression. The outcome of these forces is tissue deformation in the shape of elongation, compression, shearing, bending and torsion, or any combination of these structural changes. Stretching in all its forms, whether active or passive, relies primarily on tension loading (Fig. 6.11).

When tension load is applied by stretching there is counter-resistance from the underlying tissues. This resistance tends to change in character as the loading forces increase.[14,15] It can be felt by stretching the index finger into extension. At the resting angle of the joint the tissues are slack and there is little resistance to the stretch. This is represented by the toe region on the force–elongation curve (Fig. 6.12).[43,44] Within this range there is no true elongation of the fibres. The observed length change is similar to pulling a slack rope into tension. It will just flatten it. As the stretching increases beyond the toe region the resistance in the tissues will rise and they will feel more bouncy. This range is called the *elastic region*. Further stretching beyond this range will bring the tissues to the *plastic region*, where there is a distinct barrier-like resistance and the experience of discomfort/pain. In this range there is progressive tissue damage that starts as microtears and that can develop into full rupture if the force exceeds the tissue's tensile strength.[14,45] The end-elastic-/-plastic range can vary considerably between different tissues and their location in the body.[14,46–49]

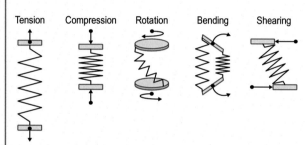

FIGURE 6.11 Tissue loading. Stretching relies on tension loading, which also takes place during rotation, bending and shearing loading.

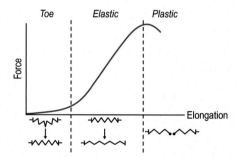

FIGURE 6.12 The force–elongation curve.

REFERENCES

1. Arampatzis A, Peper A, Bierbaum S, et al. Plasticity of human Achilles tendon mechanical and morphological properties in response to cyclic strain. J Biomech 2010;43(16):3073–9.
2. Muijka M, Padilla S. Muscular characteristics of detraining in humans. Med Sci Sports Exerc 2001;333:1297–303.
3. Maund E, Craig D, Suekarran S, et al. Management of frozen shoulder: a systematic review and cost-effectiveness analysis. Health Technol Assess 2012;16(11):1–264.
4. Tulchin K, Orendurff M, Karol L. The effects of surface slope on multi-segment foot kinematics in healthy adults. Gait Posture 2010;32(4):446–50.
5. Leroux A, Fung J, Barbeau H. Postural adaptation to walking on inclined surfaces. I. Normal strategies. Gait Posture 2002;15(1):64–74.
6. Cyron BM, Hutton WC. The tensile strength of the capsular ligaments of the apophyseal joints. J Anat 1981;132(Pt 1): 145–50.
7. Nilsson J, Thorstensson A. Ground reaction forces at different speeds of human walking and running. Acta Physiol Scand 1989;136(2):217–27.

8. Ramey MR, Williams KR. Ground reaction forces in the triple jump. J Appl Biomech 1985;1(3):233–9.

9. Magnusson SP, Simonsen EB, Aagaard P, et al. Viscoelastic response to repeated static stretching in the human hamstring muscle. Scand J Med Sci Sports 1995;5(6):342–7.

10. Magnusson SP, Simonsen EB, Aagaard P, et al. Contraction specific changes in passive torque in human skeletal muscle. Acta Physiol Scand 1995;155(4):377–86.

11. Magnusson SP, Simonsen EB, Dyhre-Poulsen P, et al. Viscoelastic stress relaxation during static stretch in human skeletal muscle in the absence of EMG activity. Scand J Med Sci Sports 1996;6(6):323–8.

12. Magnusson SP. Passive properties of human skeletal muscle during stretch maneuvers: a review. Scand J Med Sci Sports 1998;8(2):65–77.

13. Magnusson SP, Aagard P, Simonsen E, et al. A biomechanical evaluation of cyclic and static stretch in human skeletal muscle. Int J Sports Med 1998;19(5):310–16.

14. Carlstedt CA, Nordin M. Biomechanics of tendons and ligaments. In: Nordin M, Frankel VH, editors. Basic biomechanics of the musculoskeletal system. London: Lea & Febiger; 1989:698–738.

15. Zachazewski JE. Improving flexibility. In: Rosemary M, Scully RM, Barnes R, editors. Physical therapy. London: JB Lippincott; 1989.

16. Hukins DWL, Kirby MC, Sikoryn TA, et al. Comparison of structure, mechanical properties, and function of lumbar spinal ligaments. Spine 1990;15(8):787–95.

17. Hargens AR, Akeson WH. Stress effects on tissue nutrition and viability. In: Hargens AR, editor. Tissue nutrition and viability. New York: Springer; 1986.

18. Jamison CE, Marangoni RD, Glaser AA. Viscoelastic properties of soft tissue by discrete model characterization. J Biomech 1968;1:33–46.

19. Taylor DC, Dalton JD, Seaber AV, et al. Viscoelastic properties of muscle–tendon units: the biomechanical effects of stretching. Am J Sports Med 1990;18(3):300–9.

20. Esposito F, Limonta E, Cè E. Passive stretching effects on electromechanical delay and time course of recovery in human skeletal muscle: new insights from an electromyographic and mechanomyographic combined approach. Eur J Appl Physiol 2010;111(3):485–95.

21. LaBan MM. Collagen tissue: implication of its response to stress in vitro. Arch Phys Med Rehabil 1962;43:461–6.

22. Dunn MG, Silver FH. Viscoelastic behaviour of human connective tissues: relative contribution of viscous and elastic components. Connect Tissue Res 1983;12:59–70.

23. Ryan ED, Herda TJ, Costa PB, et al. Viscoelastic creep in the human skeletal muscle–tendon unit. Eur J Appl Physiol 2010;108(1):207–11.

24. Ryan ED, Herda TJ, Costa PB, et al. Dynamics of viscoelastic creep during repeated stretches. Scand J Med Sci Sports 2012;22(2):179–84.

25. Muraki T, Yamamoto N, Berglund LJ, et al. The effect of cyclic loading simulating oscillatory joint mobilization on the posterior capsule of the glenohumeral joint: a cadaveric study. Orthop Sports Phys Ther 2011;41(5):311–18.

26. Mitchell UH, Myrer JW, Hopkins JT, et al. Acute stretch perception alteration contributes to the success of the PNF "contract–relax" stretch. J Sport Rehabil 2007;16(2):85–92.

27. Duong B, Low M, Moseley AM, et al. Time course of stress relaxation and recovery in human ankles. Clin Biomech 2001;16(7):601–7.

28. Black JD, Stevens ED. Passive stretching does not protect against acute contraction-induced injury in mouse EDL muscle. J Muscle Res Cell Motil 2001;22(4):301–10.

29. Grigg NL, Wearing SC, Smeathers JE. Eccentric calf muscle exercise produces a greater acute reduction in Achilles tendon thickness than concentric exercise. Br J Sports Med 2009;43(4):280–3.

30. Chaudhry H, Bukiet B, Findley T. Mathematical analysis of applied loads on skeletal muscles during manual therapy. J Am Osteopath Assoc 2008;108(12):680–8.

31. Noyes FR, DeLucas JL, Torvik PJ. Biomechanics of anterior cruciate ligament failure: an analysis of strain-rate sensitivity and mechanisms of failure in primates. J Bone Joint Surg Am 1974;56(2):236–53.

32. Roberts JM, Wilson K. Effect of stretching duration on active and passive range of motion in the lower extremity. Br J Sports Med 1999;33(4):259–63.
33. Warren CG, Lehman F, Koblanski JN. Heat and stretch procedure: an evaluation using rat tail tendon. Arch Phys Med Rehabil 1976;57:122–6.
34. Light KE, Nuzik S, Personius W. Low load prolonged stretch vs. high load brief stretch in treating knee contractures. Phys Ther 1984;64:330–3.
35. Threlkeld J. The effects of manual therapy on connective tissue. Phys Ther 1992;72:893–902.
36. Diercks RL, Stevens M. Gentle thawing of the frozen shoulder: a prospective study of supervised neglect versus intensive physical therapy in seventy-seven patients with frozen shoulder syndrome followed up for two years. J Shoulder Elbow Surg 2004;13(5):499–502.
37. Loew M, Heichel TO, Lehner B. Intraarticular lesions in primary frozen shoulder after manipulation under general anesthesia. J Shoulder Elbow Surg 2005;14(1):16–21.
38. Cuff DJ, Pupello DR. Prospective randomized study of arthroscopic rotator cuff repair using an early versus delayed postoperative physical therapy protocol. J Shoulder Elbow Surg 2012;21(11):1450–5.
39. Lee BG, Cho NS, Rhee YG. Effect of two rehabilitation protocols on range of motion and healing rates after arthroscopic rotator cuff repair: aggressive versus limited early passive exercises. Arthroscopy 2012;28(1):34–42.
40. Meijer HJ, Rijkelijkhuizen JM, Huijing PA. Myofascial force transmission between antagonistic rat lower limb muscles: effects of single muscle or muscle group lengthening. J Electromyogr Kinesiol 2007;17(6):698–707.
41. Huijing PA, Baan GC. Myofascial force transmission causes interaction between adjacent muscles and connective tissue: effects of blunt dissection and compartmental fasciotomy on length force characteristics of rat extensor digitorum longus muscle. Arch Physiol Biochem 2001;109(2):97–109.
42. Huijing PA. Epimuscular myofascial force transmission between antagonistic and synergistic muscles can explain movement limitation in spastic paresis. J Electromyogr Kinesiol 2007;17(6):708–24.
43. De Deyne PG. Application of passive stretch and its implications for muscle fibers. Phys Ther 2001;81(2):819–27.
44. Viidik A. Interdependence between structure and function in collagenous tissues. In: Viidik A, Vuust J, editors. Biology of collagen. London: Academic Press; 1980:257–80.
45. Tillman LJ, Cummings GS. Biology mechanisms of connective tissue mutability. In: Currier DP, Nelson RM, editors. Dynamics of human biological tissue. Philadelphia: FA Davies; 1993:1–44.
46. Viidik A. Properties of tendon and ligaments. In: Skalak R, Chien S, editors. Handbook of bioengineering. New York: McGraw-Hill; 1987.
47. Rigby BJ, Hirai N, Spikes JD. The mechanical behavior of rat tail tendon. J Gen Physiol 1959;43:265–83.
48. Rigby BJ. The effect of mechanical extension upon the thermal stability of collagen. Biochim Biophys Acta 1964;79:634–6.
49. Leonard TR, Joumaa V, Herzog W. An activatable molecular spring reduces muscle tearing during extreme stretching. J Biomech 2010;43(15):3063–6.

CHAPTER 7

Exposure and Scheduling the ROM Challenge

Recently, I was standing on a beach and observing the wide range of sports activities that individuals were undertaking, in particular their warm-up routines. Whether they were about to run, swim or surf they all exhibited a similar warm-up behaviour. For a brief period, lasting no more than a few seconds, they stretched specific body areas. Further down the beach were a couple of people practising yoga. Their activity was strikingly different. Their movements were slow and, once in position, they sustained it for periods that ran into minutes. Presumably, both groups aimed to achieve a similar goal of maintaining or improving agility. Yet, increased flexibility is more likely to occur in one training condition than in the other, but which is it, and what is the optimum exposure for stretching?

This chapter explores the scheduling factor of the range of movement (ROM) challenge: the *duration* (single session), *frequency* (how often repeated) and *time span* (weeks/months), collectively termed here *exposure*. It will aim to provide answers to commonly raised question about the scheduling of stretching:

- What is the optimum duration for ROM challenges?
- How often should ROM challenges be repeated?
- Can clinical stretching or exercise provide sufficient exposure?
- How does scheduling of stretching change in the presence of pathology?
- Is there a scheduling difference between traditional and functional stretching approaches?

DURATION OF CHALLENGE

The scheduling of the ROM challenge depends largely on the intrinsic physiological processes that underlie adaptation. From a physiological perspective there is probably some ideal frequency and duration that would optimize mechanotransduction. However, this quantity is currently indefinable, partly because of the lack of research but also because of the numerous extrinsic influences that can affect this process, such as the nature and extent of the ROM pathology, the type of tissue affected and metabolic factors.

Currently, most of the information about scheduling of stretching is derived from studies of healthy young individuals. Many of the studies used passive stretching approaches, with a duration ranging from 6 to 60 seconds often quoted as being the most effective.[1–8] In the hamstrings, a daily episode of stretching for 30 seconds was found to be more effective than 15 seconds. However, there are no significant differences between stretches lasting 30 and 60 seconds,[3,4] implying that the most effective duration is about 30 seconds. This has become the unofficial duration standard for passive stretching; well, at least for the hamstring muscles.[9] Interestingly, increasing the stretching duration to 30 minutes per day, over several weeks, fails to provide any additional ROM gains.[10–12]

The 30-second duration creates a paradox. It implies that yoga practitioners and dancers might be wasting valuable training time. According to research, 30 seconds should suffice. Yet, runners who stretch for short periods are rarely able to perform the agility feats associated with flexibility training. Perhaps for adaptive changes we need to look at longer duration and extended time spans – scheduling practices that are observed in flexibility training. So the relationship between stretching exposure and gains in flexibility remains unresolved in healthy individuals. But the important question here is what happens to the stretching exposure in the presence of a ROM pathology? Does 30 seconds suffice or does it need to be raised considerably?

Duration in the presence of ROM pathology

It seems that, in the presence of pathology, the duration of stretching has to increase dramatically. It was demonstrated that 6–12 hours of daily splinting is required to overcome flexion contractures in the proximal interphalangeal joint after surgery, and more days spent in the cast resulted in greater ROM improvements (60° at 3 days and 106° at 6 days).[13,14] Another study suggested that 8–12 hours per day for 8 weeks are necessary to effectively overcome similar contractures.[15] This phenomenon was also demonstrated in frozen shoulder, in which maximizing the total time spent at end-ranges tends to improve ROM.[16] In patients with contractures due to central nervous system damage, it is estimated that over 6 hours of daily stretching would be required to improve ROM.[17,18] Several studies have explored shorter duration in patients with spinal cord injuries. ROM challenges were applied daily to the ankle for 30 minutes, over time spans of 4, 6 and 12 weeks using either passive stretching or static standing on a wedge.[10,19,20] ROM improvements were not observed in any of these studies.

These studies suggest that, in the presence of pathology, ROM challenges may have to occupy up to half of the person's waking day, which of course is unattainable unless splints are used. Even if these studies overestimated the stretching duration by 2–3 times we would still be unable to fulfil this exposure quota. Is there a solution?

Competition in ROM adaptation

Perhaps we should look at the exposure component in a different way altogether, and consider that ROM loss and recovery represent a competition in adaptation between the pathological process that maintains the condition and the ROM challenges that counteract it (Fig. 7.1).

As discussed previously, musculoskeletal adaptation tends to be specific to support movement efficiency and efficacy. Given two competing environments or training regimes, adaptation is likely to occur in the one the individual is most exposed to. This is why body-builders will find yoga difficult to perform and vice versa. It is also why those who train for flexibility need extensive stretching exposure to compete with the adaptation imposed by their daily activities. Hence, dancers seem to be in a constant state of stretching (I have seen a dancer sitting in a side-split at an air terminal while waiting for a flight, and the flight was delayed!). The question is what happens to this competition when an individual has some pathological condition which is competing with the ROM challenges?

Let us re-examine the post-surgical studies which suggest that several hours of daily splinting are required to overcome contractures. This can be viewed as a competition in adaptation between the post-surgical pathology that maintains the tissue shortening and the splinting that promotes tissue elongation/

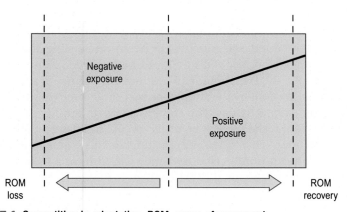

FIGURE 7.1 Competition in adaptation. ROM, range of movement.

Table 7.1 All approaches that are dependent on the therapist's assistance are unlikely to provide sufficient duration and repetition for range of movement (ROM) adaptation. However, even managed recovery behaviour may fail because of lack of adherence by the patient

	Management/ROM challenge	Does it provide enough repetition/exposure?	
Functional	Recovery behaviour	Yes	Most effective
	Managed recovery behaviour	Yes	
	Assisted recovery behaviour (functional stretching)	No	
Extra-functional	Ballistic stretching	No	
	Dynamic stretching	No	
	Muscle energy techniques	No	
	Passive stretching	No	
	Spinal manipulation	No	
	Traction	No	
	Articulation	No	
	Harmonic	No	
	Strain counter-strain	No	
	Cranial	No	Least effective

extensibility. Since the pathology that maintains the shortening is present for 24 hours per day, it is likely to win this one-sided competition, unless the duration of ROM challenge is increased dramatically. As discussed above, this would be almost impossible to attain clinically or even by exercise, so is there some other practical solution?

The solution is to tilt the competition in favour of the ROM challenge. This can be achieved by making the ROM challenges a part of the person's habitual daily activities. For example, while writing this chapter, an elderly patient consulted me about a severe shoulder sprain that took place 2 weeks previously. During that period, the patient kept her arm in a sling and close to her body at all times, which resulted in a rapid loss of glenohumeral ROM (see fear avoidance, Ch. 11). Her shoulder ROM increased dramatically, and within days of the initial session, by the simple instruction to keep the arm away from the body during daily activities. The emphasis was to amplify daily tasks that promote such ROM challenges as often as possible over behaviour that favoured shortening. This does not exclude the use of specific exercises; however, from an exposure perspective, they would have a lower therapeutic value than persistent functional ROM challenges (Table 7.1).

A competition in adaptation also means that ROM rehabilitation is more likely to succeed in self-limiting conditions (as the "negative" competition is gradually receding); it will have to be permanently maintained in persistent

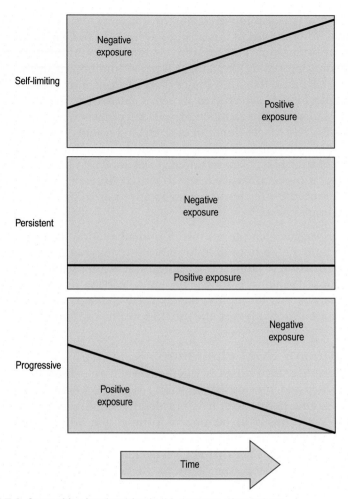

FIGURE 7.2 Competition in adaptation in the presence of pathology.

conditions ("negative" competition maintained) and ineffective in progressive conditions in which the "negative" competition is increasing (Fig. 7.2).

Ratio between maintaining and recuperating signals

A competition in adaptation suggests that there is an ideal ratio between the duration of ROM challenge and the behaviour that maintains the ROM loss.

In animal studies even short periods of passive stretching have been shown to compete with the deleterious effects of immobilization. In one of the studies the animals' limbs were immobilized in a shortened position using a sports tape.[21] Daily, the tape was removed and the limb was placed in the lengthened position and immobilized in this position using the same taping method. The immobilization duration ranged from 15 minutes to 2 hours. At the end of the lengthening procedure the animal was re-immobilized in the shortened position. It was found that 15 minutes daily of elongation was insufficient to counteract the loss of sarcomeres in series. Increasing the duration to 30 minutes daily increased the numbers of serial sarcomeres to pre-immobilization levels. Progressively longer duration of stretching resulted in further increases in the number of serial sarcomeres. In a similar immobilization study, even 15 minutes of stretching every second day was shown to be sufficient for normalizing the ratio of connective tissue to muscle fibres.[22,23] Shorter durations, such as a 40-minute stretch once a week, were not sufficient to prevent the loss of serial sarcomeres.[24]

These studies suggest that the competition in adaptation does not have to be in the same ratio, i.e. an hour of immobilization does not have to be matched by an equal duration of elongation. Clinically, it is impossible to estimate this ratio. The simple solution is for the patient to use the recovery behaviour as frequently as possible during the day. Is there a danger of overexposure to ROM challenges? Probably not: the more exposure, the better.

Termination of ROM challenge

One question that often arises is whether regular stretching has any lasting effects. As discussed previously, stretching is not a physiological necessity (Ch. 1); from this perspective, it is mostly an extra-functional pursuit. This means that stretching is in permanent competition with daily movement needs. In normal healthy individuals, cessation of regular stretching would result in rapid return to the physiological default. That is why people/athletes who stretch can never stop. The return to the default is very rapid upon cessation of stretching. It was shown that a break of 4 weeks completely reversed the gains of 6 weeks of stretching.[25] I experienced this as a yoga teacher. Seven years of gains in flexibility were almost totally abolished within several months of cessation of practice.

In individuals with pathological ROM losses, early termination of ROM challenges may result in a longer recovery time by tilting the competition in favour of the pathology. However, as the condition is improving the balance in the competition tilts towards the positive exposures (as the individual is spending longer duration in functional activities that challenge their losses, Fig. 7.1). These are often sufficient to eradicate the remaining ROM loss and also to maintain permanently the ROM improvements (*functional loading maintains functional ROM*; Ch. 5). This means that treatment can be terminated when the patient returns to functionality or is able to self-maintain recovery behaviour. This principle was discussed in Chapter 2.

SCHEDULING IN FUNCTIONAL AND EXTRA-FUNCTIONAL APPROACHES

We have still not been able to define the optimal duration and frequency of stretching. This is partly because we are looking at scheduling in two very different stretching approaches: functional and extra-functional.

In an extra-functional approach the challenges are distinct and dissimilar to normal daily activities, and as such they require specific set-aside times. Therefore, the duration and frequency of exposure have to be quantified clearly. However, there is a problem with quantifying. There are wide differences between individuals and the pathological processes that underlie their ROM loss. As a consequence, it would be almost impossible to reach a universal scheduling truth. Perhaps this is why, after half a century of research on stretching, we are still trying to solve the scheduling conundrum.

In a functional approach the scheduling is simpler. The challenges closely resemble the daily tasks and therefore there is no boundary between "exercising" and daily activities. There is no distinct set-aside exercise time and therefore quantifying the exposure is not essential. Here, the patient is given the simple advice to amplify certain daily activities as often as possible. A patient with limited stride length can be instructed to walk with a wider gait, as often as possible throughout the day. If they adhere to this simple management it could result in 10,000 repetitions of hip stretching per day. It is simple and therapeutically economical.

A note on control of active ROM and task exposure

Increasing the daily exposure to a functional task is well supported by motor control research. It is well established that regular practice is a key training condition for motor learning/adaptation.[26] Frequent and regular practice plays a crucial role in the transformation of motor experiences from short- to long-term memory.[27-30] Frequent practice of a task reduces the error and strengthens the neural networks that control that particular task.[31,32] Increasing the task exposure is therefore important for recovering the control of active ROM.

From a motor control perspective it is also difficult to quantify the optimal exposure to the task. Research in this area suggests exposure that contains thousands to several millions repetition.[33] This supports the functional message that management should be expanded to encompass habitual daily activities in which the affected tasks are often repeated.

Although motor recovery shares the same neurophysiological mechanisms as motor learning, there is an important difference here. In ROM recovery the patient is not a learner. Most often they have lost the capacity to execute the movement for central or musculoskeletal reasons, rather than "unlearning" it.

This means that they do not have to learn the movement from scratch but to reorganize it optimally for functional use. It may also mean that the exposure to the ROM challenge can be lower than the one needed for learning a novel task. However, this motor optimization/reorganization still relies on numerous repetitions. How many? We do not know, but probably a lot.

ADHERENCE TO THE PROGRAMME

A functional approach that promotes recovery behaviour is in essence a self-care programme which engages the patient's self-efficacy capacity and autonomy.[34] Self-care is essential for maintaining the rehabilitation programme; in particular because ROM recovery is expected to be in time scales of weeks or months. The success of self-care is highly dependent on the patient's adherence to the programme. Yet, it is well established that adherence tends to be low at best and reduces very rapidly.[35,36] So when we look at the exposure component we also have to consider the factors that could help to sustain the treatment programme.

Generally, attitudes, beliefs and self-motivation determine exercise compliance and adherence.[34,37-40] Included is the person's belief in their ability to succeed in a particular situation (self-efficacy),[41] enjoyment of physical activity, support from others,[39] positive beliefs concerning the benefits of physical activity,[42] and a lack of perceived barriers to being physically active.[37,42] These factors can be translated into attainable management strategies:

■ **Keep the patient (positively) informed** about the condition and why their participation can help adaptation.[42-44] Often I will describe the principle of recovery behaviour and a bit about how the body converts physical activity into structural changes in the tissues. Adherence is also improved by information that empowers the patient (Ch. 11).[45-47]
■ **Identify patient-centred goals.**[42] Focus on goals that are important to the patient, rather than on clinical goals. This will help to motivate the patient to maintain the ROM management.[48,49]
■ **Develop ROM challenges not exercise**. I tend to use the phrase "daily challenges" rather than "exercise", particularly with individuals who are exercise-shy. The notion of exercise is often associated with activities that require set-aside time, specialized equipment and are carried out in a dedicated location such as a gym.[50] These elements tend to shift the locus of care further away from the individual's immediate environment. On the other hand, some patients need organized exercise regimes with defined daily schedules.
■ **Make the challenges readily available.**[48,51] The ROM challenges are often amplification of end-range movements encountered during normal daily activities. Keep the challenges as close as possible to the patient's func-

tional repertoire, incorporated into their home, work and recreational activities. This approach brings the care within reach of the individual's environment and is therefore more likely to contribute to adherence.[34,48]

- **Keep it simple.** Avoid complex management protocols or exercise. Simple routines tend to increase compliance.[52] It has been found that patients may have difficulties in recalling information, in particular statements that contain instructions and advice.[53] So keeping it short and simple and repeating the message in subsequent sessions could be helpful.[42] Furthermore, it was found that patients who understand the management concepts are able to transfer and modify these principles to fit their lifestyles; they were able to devise their own exercises and further personalize the management of their condition.[39]

- **Provide ongoing support and feedback.**[42] **And make it fun.** The element of enjoyment is also important for exercise adherence. It is useful to create a wish-list of activities that the patient enjoys and would like to return to. Strive to develop ROM challenges within these activities.[39]

SUMMARY

- This chapter explored the exposure and scheduling of the ROM challenge: duration, frequency and time span
- Currently, there are no clear guidelines on the scheduling of ROM challenges
- ROM rehabilitation represents a competition in adaptation between the pathological process that maintains the condition and the ROM challenge that counteracts it
- It is estimated that in the presence of pathology the daily ROM challenges should be for several hours
- A functional approach aims to tilt the competition in favour of physical environments or behaviour that drive ROM recovery. This can be achieved by incorporating the ROM challenge into the daily activities
- Long-term maintenance of the ROM rehabilitation programme is dependent on the patient's self-care ability
- Adherence to the programme may be helped by positive information about the condition, identifying goals that are important to the patient and simplifying and making the challenges readily available
- Adherence means that the patient has a shared responsibility/role in their recovery
- Message to the patient – "what ever you do, do more"

REFERENCES

1. Taylor DC, Dalton JD, Seaber AV, et al. Viscoelastic properties of muscle–tendon units: the biomechanical effects of stretching. Am J Sports Med 1990;18(3):300–9.

2. McNair PJ, Dombroski EW, Hewson DJ, et al. Stretching at the ankle joint: viscoelastic responses to holds and continuous passive motion. Med Sci Sports Exerc 2001;33(3):354–8.

3. Bandy WD, Irion JM, Briggler M. The effect of time and frequency of static stretching on flexibility of the hamstring muscles. Phys Ther 1997;77(10):1090–6.

4. Bandy WD, Irion JM. The effect of time on static stretch on the flexibility of the hamstring muscles. Phys Ther 1994;74(9):845–50.

5. Magnusson SP, Simonsen EB, Aagaard P, et al. Viscoelastic response to repeated static stretching in the human hamstring muscle. Scand J Med Sci Sports 1995;5(6):342–7.

6. Magnusson SP, Simonsen EB, Aagaard P, et al. Contraction specific changes in passive torque in human skeletal muscle. Acta Physiol Scand 1995;155(4):377–86.

7. Magnusson SP. Passive properties of human skeletal muscle during stretch maneuvers: a review. Scand J Med Sci Sports 1998;8(2):65–77.

8. Roberts JM, Wilson K. Effect of stretching duration on active and passive range of motion in the lower extremity. Br J Sports Med 1999;33(4):259–63.

9. Decoster LC. Effects of hamstring stretching on range of motion: a systematic review updated. Athlet Train Sports Health Care 2009;1(5):209–13.

10. Harvey LA, Byak AJ, Ostrovskaya M, et al. Randomised trial of the effects of four weeks of daily stretch on extensibility of hamstring muscles in people with spinal cord injuries. Aust J Physiother 2009;2003;49(3):176–81.

11. Folpp H, Deall S, Harvey LA, et al. Can apparent increases in muscle extensibility with regular stretch be explained by changes in tolerance to stretch? Aust J Physiother 2006;52(1):45–50.

12. Ben M, Harvey LA. Regular stretch does not increase muscle extensibility: a randomized controlled trial. Scand J Med Sci Sports 2010;20(1):136–44.

13. Flowers KR, LaStayo P. Effect of total end range time on improving passive range of motion. J Hand Ther 1994;7(3):150–7.

14. Glasgow C, Wilton J, Tooth L. Optimal daily total end range time for contracture: resolution in hand splinting. J Hand Ther 2003;16(3):207–18.

15. Prosser R. Splinting in the management of proximal interphalangeal joint flexion contracture. J Hand Ther 1996;9(4):378–86.

16. Dempsey AL, Mills T, Karsch RM, et al. Maximizing total end range time is safe and effective for the conservative treatment of frozen shoulder patients. Am J Phys Med Rehabil 2011;90(9):738–45.

17. Tardieu C, Lespargot A, Tabary C, et al. For how long must the soleus muscle be stretched each day to prevent contracture? Dev Med Child Neurol 1988;30:3–10.

18. Hufschmidt A, Mauritz KH. Chronic transformation of muscle in spasticity: a peripheral contribution to increased tone. J Neurol Neurosurg Psychiatry 1985;48(7):676–85.

19. Harvey LA, Batty J, Crosbie J, et al. A randomized trial assessing the effects of 4 weeks of daily stretching on ankle mobility in patients with spinal cord injuries. Arch Phys Med Rehabil 2000;81(10):1340–7.

20. Ben M, Harvey L, Denis S, et al. Does 12 weeks of regular standing prevent loss of ankle mobility and bone mineral density in people with recent spinal cord injuries? Aust J Physiother 2005;51(4):251–6.

21. Williams PE. Use of intermittent stretch in the prevention of serial sarcomere loss in immobilised muscle. Ann Rheum Dis 1990;49:316–17.

22. Williams PE. Effect of intermittent stretch on immobilised muscle. Ann Rheum Dis 1988;47:1014–16.

23. Williams PE. The morphological basis of increased stiffness of rabbit tibialis anterior during surgical limb-lengthening. J Anat 1998;193:131–8.

24. Gomes AR, Coutinho EL, França CN, et al. Effect of one stretch a week applied to the immobilized soleus muscle on rat muscle fiber morphology. Braz J Med Biol Res 2004;37(10):1473–80.

25. Willy RW, Kyle BA, Moore SA, et al. Effect of cessation and resumption of static hamstring muscle stretching on joint range of motion. Orthop Sports Phys Ther 2001;31(3):138–44.

26. Lederman E. Neuromuscular rehabilitation in manual and physical therapies. Edinburgh: Elsevier; 2010.

27. Magill RA. Motor learning concepts and applications. Dubuque, IA: William C Brown; 1985.

28. Schmidt RA, Lee TD. Motor control and learning. 4th ed. Champaign, IL: Human Kinetics; 2005.

29. Fitts PM, Posner MI. Human performance. Pacific Grove, CA: Brooks/Cole; 1967.

30. Adams JA. Short-term memory for motor responses. J Exp Psychol 1966;71(2):314–18.

31. Lee TD, Swanson LR, Hall AL. What is repeated in a repetition? Effects of practice conditions on motor skill acquisition. Phys Ther 1991;71(2):150–6.

32. Khan MA, Franks IM, Goodman D. The effect of practice on the control of rapid aiming movements: evidence for an interdependency between programming and feedback processing. Q J Exp Psychol Hum Exp Psychol 1998;51A:425–44.

33. Kottke FJ, Halpern D, Easton JK, et al. The training of coordination. Arch Phys Med Rehabil 1978;59:567–72.

34. Chan DK, Lonsdale C, Ho PY, et al. Patient motivation and adherence to postsurgery rehabilitation exercise recommendations: the influence of physiotherapists' autonomy-supportive behaviors. Arch Phys Med Rehabil 2009;90(12):1977–82.

35. Häkkinen A, Kautiainen H, Hannonen P, et al. Strength training and stretching versus stretching only in the treatment of patients with chronic neck pain: a randomized one-year follow-up study. Clin Rehabil 2008;22(7):592–600.

36. Jordan JL, Holden MA, Mason EE, et al. Interventions to improve adherence to exercise for chronic musculoskeletal pain in adults. Cochrane Database Syst Rev 2010;1:CD005956.

37. Schneider RC, Aiken FA. Environmental and activity characteristics on exercise adherence. ICHPERD-SD J Res 2008;3(1):51–6.

38. Minor MA, Brown JD. Exercise maintenance of persons with arthritis after participation in a class experience. Health Educ Behav 1993;20(1):83–95.

39. Jolly K, Taylor R, Lip GY, et al. The Birmingham Rehabilitation Uptake Maximisation Study (BRUM). Home-based compared with hospital-based cardiac rehabilitation in a multi-ethnic population: cost-effectiveness and patient adherence. Health Technol Assess 2007;11(35):1–118.

40. Schwarzer R, et al. Social-cognitive predictors of physical exercise adherence: three longitudinal studies in rehabilitation. Health Psychol 2008;27(1, Suppl):S54–63.

41. Bandura A. Self-efficacy in changing societies. Cambridge, UK: Cambridge University Press; 1995.

42. Sluijs EM, Kok GJ, van der Zee J. Correlates of exercise compliance in physical therapy. Phys Ther 1993;73(11):771–82.

43. McCall LA, Ginis KAM. The effects of message framing on exercise adherence and health beliefs among patients in a cardiac rehabilitation program. J Appl Biobehav Res 2004;9(2):122–35.

44. Henrotin YE, Cedraschi C, Duplan B, et al. Information and low back pain management: a systematic review. Spine 2006;31(11):E326–34.

45. Burton AK, Waddell G, Tillotson KM, et al. Information and advice to patients with back pain can have a positive effect: a randomised controlled trial of a novel educational booklet in primary care. Spine 1999;24:2484–91.

46. Linton SJ, Andersson T. Can chronic disability be prevented? A randomized trial of a cognitive-behavior intervention and two forms of information for patients with spinal pain. Spine 2000;25(21):2825–31.

47. Moseley GL, Nicholas MK, Hodges PW. A randomized controlled trial of intensive neurophysiology education in chronic low back pain. Clin J Pain 2004;20(5):324–30.

48. Evenson K, Fleury J. Barriers to outpatient cardiac rehabilitation participation and adherence. J Cardiopulm Rehabil 2000;20(4):241–6.

49. Locke EA. Toward a theory of task motivation incentives. J Organ Behav Hum Perform 1966;3:157–89.

50. Hassett LM, Tate RL, Moseley AM, et al. Injury severity, age and pre-injury exercise history predict adherence to a home-based exercise programme in adults with traumatic brain injury. Brain Inj 2011;25(7–8):698–706.
51. Jackson L, Leclerc J, Erskine Y, et al. Getting the most out of cardiac rehabilitation: a review of referral and adherence predictors. Heart 2005;91:10–14.
52. Dolan-Mullen P, Green LW, Persinger GS. Clinical trials of patient education for chronic conditions: a comparative meta-analysis of intervention types. Prev Med 1985;14:753–81.
53. Ice R. Long term compliance. Phys Ther 1985;65:1832–9.

CHAPTER 8

Rehabilitating the Active ROM: Neuromuscular Consideration

Imagine a common clinical scenario in which a treatment is about to commence for the stiff, non-painful frozen shoulder. Several questions come to mind as we plan the management. Should we begin treatment with passive stretching and later add the active challenges; start both simultaneously; or not bother with passive stretching? When using an active approach, should the movement be broken up to focus on specific shoulder or scapular muscles or focus on whole arm movements? What kind of active movement should be used, functional, extra-functional? Above all, what exactly is being rehabilitated in the active range and is there a way of making the process more effective?

This chapter will explore the active component of range of movement (ROM) rehabilitation and will aim to provide answers to these commonly raised questions:

- What is being rehabilitated in the active ROM?
- Which elements of motor control are the targets of ROM rehabilitation?
- Should rehabilitation be of part or whole movement?
- Should ROM rehabilitation be sequenced from passive to active rehabilitation or should they be concurrent?
- Can passive approaches help recover motor control?
- How does focus of attention influence recovery of active ROM?
- What is rehabilitated in task-specific rehabilitation?

GOALS AND FOCUS OF ATTENTION

Curiously, what we focus on while we train or move can influence learning and the efficiency and effectiveness of our movements. When we observe human movement, a large selection of this repertoire is directed towards external goals: to reach for a cup, hit a ball or walk across a room. Movement goals are rarely internal to specific body parts; we do not set out to move our limbs, joints or contract specific muscles.[1] Whether the focus of attention is external or internal has important implications for ROM rehabilitation.

101

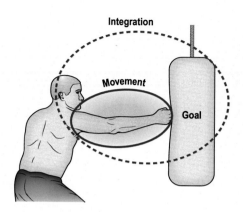

FIGURE 8.1 The movement that typifies a task is integrated with its goals.

For an outsider observing a person performing a task, say lifting a cup, the action can be broken into two components (Fig. 8.1): the movement that typifies the task (unique arm movement) and the goal of this movement (to lift the cup). However, this separation is artificial. In most activities the movement and its goals are a unified response and not separate entities.[2] When we are learning a new task the movement and its goal are integrated and represented internally as images of the goal. The intention to attain the goal triggers the execution of the associated movement, including all the anticipatory postural adjustments that precede it.[3–6]

The integration of the movement with its goals and the direction of focus create an order of effect in ROM management (Fig. 8.2). Movement, motor

Nature of ROM challenge	Focus of attention	Therapeutic effectiveness
Goal movement (movement + goal)	External focus	Most effective
Movement only	Internal focus (correctness of movement)	
Part of the movement sequence	Internal focus	
Fragmented movement	Extreme internal focus	Least effective

FIGURE 8.2 Hierarchy in range of movement (ROM) challenge. Motor learning and performance are enhanced by challenges that integrate the movement and its goals.

learning and recovery are most effective when the focus of attention is directed towards external goals, i.e. training or rehabilitation that engages this natural integration.[7-14] Less effective is rehabilitation in which the focus is internal, on movement itself and separated from its goals. Below this level is the "extreme" internal focus in which movement itself is fragmented into smaller units to become the focus and goal of rehabilitation. Here, the focus of attention is directed towards specific muscles or joints that make up the movement.

Internal focus is often represented in rehabilitation as "correctness of movement", where faults in movement are identified and corrected. It can have a negative or positive influence on movement depending on the the skill level of the individual. It tends to degrade task performance if the person is already skilled in the task. It has a positive effect when the individual is learning a novel task. However, in ROM rehabilitation the individual is often experienced in the task but is unable to perform it because of physical/motor constraints. Hence, external focus is more effective, whereas internal focus is mostly superfluous and may even be detrimental in ROM rehabilitation. Extreme internal focus is often represented in ROM rehabilitation by contract–relax methods or by muscle-by-muscle or muscle chain rehabilitation. From a motor control perspective it is considered to be the least effective form of training and rehabilitation.

The evidence to support the use of goal-orientated movement in rehabilitation is derived from focus-of-attention studies.[7-14] In these studies individuals are instructed to focus either on the goal/outcome of the movement (external focus) or on a particular part of the body (internal focus). It was demonstrated that even simple tasks such as biceps curls are executed more effectively and efficiently under external focus (concentrating on the curl bar) rather than internal focus (concentrating on the biceps muscle or movement of the arm). The group using internal focus had lower electromyography (EMG) activity than the external focus group, although both groups were lifting the same weight.[15,16] In a study of force production in the leg, subjects were instructed to either "push your foot against the plate" (external focus) or "push with the muscle of the calf" (internal focus).[17] Using external focus resulted in less error in force production, more efficient co-contraction and optimized EMG activity. Similarly, in studies on jump height, subjects were instructed to focus externally on the goal, "concentrate on the highest rungs", or internally, "concentrate on your fingers". The external focus group demonstrated increased jump height and greater force production while exhibiting lower EMG activity.[18,19] The effects of focus of attention have also been observed in trunk muscle activation during sudden load change. In this study, a load was applied to the subject's back and then suddenly removed. Throughout that task subjects were instructed to resist the load either by their naturally chosen manner (external focus) or by abdominal bracing (internal focus).[20] The naturally selected manner resulted in more effective muscle recruitment patterns of the spine. Conscious, voluntary overdriving of this natural pattern resulted in unbalanced muscular activation patterns and increased the loading on the spine to dangerously high levels.

Overall, the studies on focus of attention demonstrate that focusing on the outcome of the movement rather than on the body and its workings enables the individual to produce greater peak forces, execute faster movement, and increase joint movement accuracy with less muscular activity.[14,15,18,19] External, goal-focused training engages the individual in whole movement patterns that promote movement economy.[17] It also optimizes motor learning by promoting movement automatism earlier in the training as well as facilitating transfer of learning to novel situations (Ch. 5).[18,21] These studies suggest that an external focus of attention is a more effective strategy for rehabilitating the active ROM.

External–internal focus in ROM rehabilitation

The difference between external and internal focus approaches has important practical manifestations in shaping the ROM challenges. This can be exemplified by flexion rehabilitation of the shoulder. In the internal focus approach, the patient is instructed to contract their anterior deltoid, elongate the pectorals, stabilize the scapula and so on. In the external goal approach, the patient is instructed simply to reach with their hand to the ceiling. The outcome is likely to be the same for both approaches – a full flexion range. However, in the goal approach the individual is training in more efficient movement patterns which are within task. This raises the potential for transfer of training gains from the rehabilitation to functional activities (Ch. 5).[7-14] Furthermore, external focus is clinically more economical. Minimum instruction is producing a maximum effect. The patient is not required to have any knowledge of anatomy or movement physiology; more importantly, they do not have to learn anything new. The rehabilitation is *using what the patient already knows*. In the external focus/goal approach, the patient needs only a modest training investment to recover control of the shoulder. In the internal approach the patient is required to learn a new complex movement pattern, which is less effective and efficient and which often demands greater therapist involvement and additional treatments.

Regression from goal to movement level

There are occasions when attention could regress from an external to an internal focus. Imagine a patient who has flexion contractures of the elbow. When attempting a goal movement, such as reaching, rather than extending their elbow the patient may compensate by twisting and bending forward. In this situation it could be useful to instruct the patient to focus internally, on the elbow, and attempt to straighten the arm while reaching. However, even when the rehabilitation regresses to a movement level ("keep the elbow straight") it should aim to be within the context of the overall goal ("keep you elbow straight while reaching for the cup").

There are clinical solutions to limit postural compensations and minimize the need for internal focus. In the elbow scenario above, the forward trunk movement can be restrained by instructing the patient to hold the back of the chair with the opposite arm while performing the reaching movement (Ch. 13). Another strategy is to let the patient "cheat" and bend forward, but, then, place the target even further away until forward bending is no longer possible. In both of these examples the patient will be forced to extend the elbow maximally to reach the target. A similar tactic can be used to recover flexion and abduction range in a frozen shoulder (Ch. 13). Often, a seated patient will use trunk side-bending to compensate for abduction restriction, and trunk extension to compensate for flexion restrictions. This can be overcome by placing the target further away from the body, laterally or in front, forcing the patient to execute greater shoulder abduction and flexion movements.

TASK-SPECIFIC MUSCLE RECRUITMENT

The organization of movement around its goals means that any given muscle will participate in many different tasks, rather than a specific one (Fig. 8.3).

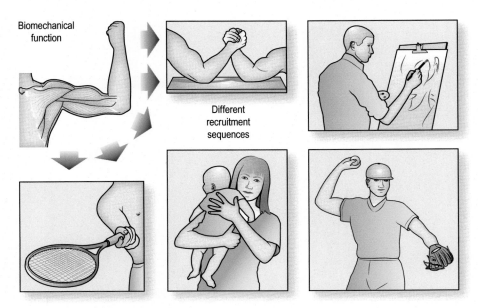

FIGURE 8.3 Same muscle, many functions.

This means that muscle recruitment is *task specific*.[22-27] Task-specific recruitment can be likened to a speaker (the muscle) through which different music tracks (motor programmes) can be played. For example, there is a completely different recruitment pattern of the trunk muscles during standing, walking, reaching to the sides, forward bending or lifting or any other imaginable movement.[26-30] We cannot claim that the spinal multifidus muscle is exclusively designed for any one of these activities (as is often claimed in many physical therapy approaches). However, we could state that its anatomical location and mechanical function mean that it has a varying role in all these movements, and many more.

Integrate or fragment?

Task-dependent muscle recruitment determines whether a movement should be rehabilitated as a whole or fragmented to smaller anatomical units (Fig. 8.4). Rehabilitating a specific muscle or muscle chain is unlikely to improve the performance or recover the control of the whole task. This is because the task determines the muscle's activation pattern and not the other way round. It would be like trying to learn a tennis serve by practising biceps activation,

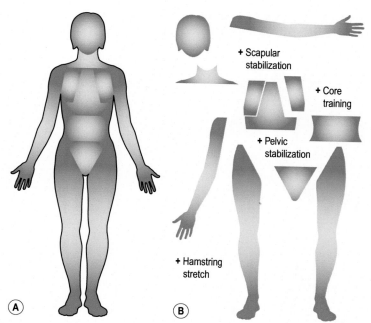

FIGURE 8.4 A. There is a whole system/person organization during movement. There are no closed or isolated muscle systems in the body. **B.** Fragmenting the body into specific anatomical/functional components does not reflect normal organization/control of movement.

Integrate   *Coordinate*
~~Fragment~~ in order to ~~integrate~~

FIGURE 8.5 Changing the old physical therapy maxim ….

triceps and then forearm control, and so on. The only way to recover normal function is to practise the task itself, during which the whole recruitment sequence is rehearsed simultaneously.

Single muscle or muscle-chain activation simply does not exist in motor organization or in the physiology of movement. ROM rehabilitation that favours movement fragmentation is more likely to improve the specific fragmented activity but not the whole movement (Fig. 8.5).[31] For example, training that improves the local power at the ankle or at the ankle and knee fails to transfer to gains in vertical jumping, although this task depends on these neuromuscular components.[31] Likewise, exercises that isolate parts of the kicking action are not recommended because they do not appear to transfer well to kicking performance; training should be of the whole kicking action.[32] It has also been demonstrated that training in isolated tasks, such as hip flexibility or trunk-strengthening activities, does not improve the economy of walking or running.[33]

Further support for whole movement training comes from the focus-of-attention studies described above. Training that promotes external focus is essentially engaging the individual in whole movement training, whereas internal focus is closely related to movement fragmentation. As discussed, external focus, goal-orientated movement provides more effective and efficient movement patterns. By normalizing the task, adaptation occurs simultaneously throughout the neuromuscular axis: centrally as motor control changes and peripherally as muscle adaptation.

If Aristotle was alive now he would have pointed out that "The task is different from the sum of its muscles and joints".

Synergy in pathology

Take a task such as a high kick. It requires an explosive shortening contraction of the hip flexors. But the success of this movement also relies on the simultaneous "explosive relaxation" and elongation of the hip extensors.[34] So muscles do not work alone but in complex synergies.

Movement synergy means that when a muscle is affected it will inevitably alter the control of all its synergists. It has been demonstrated that induced fatigue in the hamstrings will influence the control of non-exercised quadriceps.

Similarly, induced fatigue in the biceps influences triceps control.[35-37] This effect was shown to spread even to more distant synergists. For example, fatigue in quadriceps will also influence the control of the non-exercised gastrocnemius muscle.[38] So, even in pathology, muscles do not work alone but are controlled in complex synergies.

The interplay between synergists suggests that, if one muscle group is pathologically shorter, the control of all the synergists is likely to change. Imagine a clinical situation in which a patient with reduced hip ROM tries to recover the ability to perform a high kick. There are two potential therapeutic approaches: traditional fragmentation of movement, treating each loss separately, or using task-specific whole movement approaches. In the traditional approach the patient might be given hip flexor resistance exercises to improve active hip flexion and hamstring exercises to increase antagonists' extensibility. However, such fragmentation cannot capture the complex intermuscular coordination of the synergists. The pattern of recruitment during this procedure is highly dissimilar and therefore non-transferable to a high kick (see specificity and transfer of training, Ch. 5). The complexity of intermuscular coordination and its specificity to particular exercise can be resolved by simply challenging the whole movement, in the context of the goal task, i.e. practising high kicks will challenge and normalize that task.

FOCUS OF ROM REHABILITATION

We have so far identified that ROM rehabilitation should be of whole movement and practised within the context of the goal task. However, we are still left with the question of what is being rehabilitated within the task. To answer this question we need to explore what happens to the task parameters in the presence of injury and pain.

The task parameters are controlled centrally as part of normal movement organization. In the presence of injury, pain or even fear of movement the task parameters are attenuated as a protection strategy (Fig. 8.6).[39-61] This movement reorganization serves to reduce the physical stresses imposed on the injured areas. The outcome is the experience of force loss, slower movements, limitation in movement range and early onset of fatigue, which serves to reduce iteration of potentially damaging movements. This strategy is universal and can be seen throughout the body in various musculoskeletal conditions. It is a normal and advantageous motor control response; it does not represent a central pathology. The capacity for central adaptation and motor reorganization is preserved and therefore the likelihood for active ROM recovery remains high. The task parameters can also be affected by central nervous system (CNS) damage.[62-65] In these conditions central adaptive capacity is reduced and therefore the potential for ROM recovery is more limited (Ch. 3).

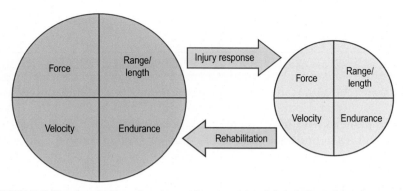

FIGURE 8.6 The organization of movement in response to injury, pain or fear of movement. The four movement parameters tend to be attenuated. One role of range of movement rehabilitation is to amplify these movement components within task challenges.

The production of force, velocity, length and endurance are also peripheral phenomena of the muscle's structure and physiology. Fortunately, by challenging the task parameter there is concurrent stimulation and adaptation of the whole neuromuscular axis, central and peripheral, motor control and muscle. They cannot be targeted individually as is sometimes believed. This means that, in ROM rehabilitation, we do not have to focus specifically on the shortened muscle. Performing a task at end-range will drive simultaneously the central and the peripheral recuperative processes.

There are other movement components that can be the focus of ROM rehabilitation such as coordination and balance. These are outside the scope of this book and can be found in Lederman.[42]

IMPORTANCE OF COGNITION

Cognition is a broad term to describe mental processes such as attention, understanding, remembering, thinking, rationalizing, memorizing, imagination, planning, decision-making and problem-solving. It has been demonstrated that these play an important role in motor learning and recovery of movement control in various musculoskeletal conditions and following CNS damage.[66–70]

Cognitive factors play an important role in ROM rehabilitation. Learning a movement pattern or recovering control requires conscious attention to particular aspects of the movement, being aware of the ranges affected and the daily tasks that could be used to challenge them.[71,72] Cognitive management also includes the patient's involvement in problem-solving, decision-making, goal-setting, planning and scheduling of practice/rehabilitation.[18,69,70,73–76] It has been shown that treatment can be more effective if these factors are an integral part of the management.[18,69,70,73–76]

The successful integration of cognitive elements in the treatment depends on the cognitive state of the patient, the therapist's awareness of their importance and effective communication but also on the therapeutic relationship between the practitioner and patient (see psychological consideration, Ch. 11). For example, patients who have cognitive losses as a result of CNS damage may have difficulties in understanding instructions or making choices. Under these circumstances, movement rehabilitation may be prolonged or impeded.

Cognition and feedback

Imagine you are learning a new task, such as a golf swing. The rate of learning and your skill of performance will partly depend on feedback from your own body and the instructor. In a similar manner, the recovery of active ROM can be enhanced or impeded by provision or withdrawal of feedback.[77–86] In ROM rehabilitation, feedback can take different forms: sensory feedback, task feedback and feedback on recovery progress.

Sensory feedback is the intrinsic, ongoing information provided from proprioceptors and other sensory modalities such as vision, auditory and vestibular (again, for full discussion, see Lederman[42]). It is a subconscious form of feedback, but it can be raised to a cognitive, conscious level by drawing attention to the body or to a particular sensory modality.[87–89] It is often used during stretching to raise awareness of tension or to promote relaxation in particular parts of the body. Although there is much interest in physical therapies in this form of feedback, it is fairly immutable to modification by physical means – you can become more aware of it but cannot change it..[42]

Task feedback is often provided by the therapist and contains information about the "correctness" of the movement ("hold the racket this way"), the movement sequences ("swing it like this") or the quality in performance ("good shot"). Sensory and task feedback are often provided as verbal instructions, visual demonstration and physical correction of movement by the therapist/ trainer.[44,90]

Generally, feedback is more effective if it promotes an active gathering of information and problem-solving by the patient.[91] For optimum learning, guidance should be kept to a minimum and rapidly reduced or fully withdrawn at the earliest opportunity.[9,68,86,92–95] Furthermore, training is found to be more effective when the feedback emphasizes successful performance and ignores less successful attempts.[19,96]

Tracking recovery progress is another important form of feedback which is usually set against specific treatment goals. Tracking can be of various treatment outcomes such as changes in ROM, pain and functional improvements.

LIMITATIONS OF EXTRA-FUNCTIONAL STRETCHING APPROACHES

So far this chapter has explored motor control and has suggested the importance of functional whole task movements. But what about other non-functional approaches? What role do they have in normalizing motor control? Do active approaches, such as muscle energy techniques (METs) and proprioceptive neuromuscular facilitation (PNF) stretching, have any role in helping the recovery of the active range? Similarly, do passive stretching approaches have any effect on motor control? To answer these questions we need to examine the physiological mechanism which these approaches purport to activate, in particular reflexive mechanisms such as autogenic inhibition and reciprocal inhibition.[97]

Motor control during active and passive stretching

Being active is essential for motor learning and recovery.[42] Movement is organized in sequences that involve afferent sensory input, central integration and an efferent motor output (Fig. 8.7).[68] During active movement this sequence is fully engaged, whereas during passive movement there is an absence of

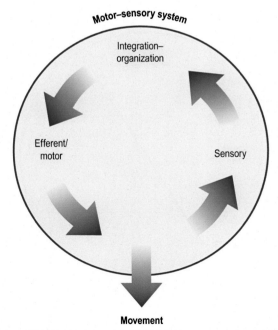

FIGURE 8.7 The organization for movement. During active movement the efferent and afferent signals are coupled.

efferent motor activity (Fig. 8.8). This efferent activity is essential for encoding the movement sequences and without it motor adaptation/learning/reorganization is unlikely to occur (with the exception of motor visualization).[98-108] Indeed, human movement and motor learning is exclusively active in nature. In comparison, passive movements are rare and are mostly associated with physical therapy.

Furthermore, during motor learning, a unique sensory image is created for that particular movement – we become familiar with what the task "feels like". Although this sensory experience will occur during both active and passive movement, it is different and likely to be non-transferable between the two (see sensory specificity, Ch. 5). The sensory experience during passive stretching will fail to match the sensory experience during a similar active movement. Another difference is that only during active movement is the sensory experience (afferent) coupled with motor processes (efferent). This sensory–motor coupling has important implications for correcting movement errors and consequently for enhancing motor learning and recovery.[109-114] This was demonstrated several decades ago in studies in which visual illusions were created by wearing special distorting lenses.[81] The ability of the subject to accurately position the arm was greatly enhanced by active (sensory–motor coupling) rather than passive (only sensory input)

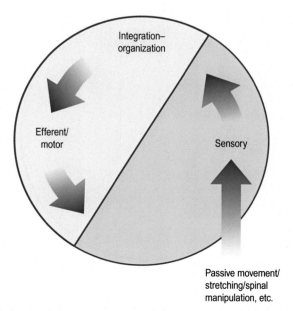

FIGURE 8.8 During passive techniques only the sensory element of the system is stimulated. There is no efferent activity and the motor–sensory coupling does not occur.

arm movement. This group of researchers concluded that an active form of movement is a prerequisite for motor learning. They stated that "active movement yields highly significant adaptive effects whereas passive movement yields either significantly less adaptation or none at all".[81]

There is also a psychological consideration in treatments that engage the individual actively. The goal of ROM rehabilitation is to return the individual to functional movement, which is active in nature. The distance between being active and proactive is very small, and, therefore, the experience of being active during the session can translate more readily into daily activities. However, the distance between being passive and proactive can be large. Treatments that are predominantly passive may set up negative therapeutic conditions in which the patient becomes uninvolved and detached – a "passive" recipient of treatment.

In summary, active ROM is unlikely to be recovered by passive stretching approaches.

Autogenic inhibition

There is a commonly held belief that stretching can reduce motor tone in a muscle by a process of autogenic inhibition.[115,116] In this model, stretching stimulates muscle–tendon receptors, resulting in inhibition of the motoneurons which supply the same muscle. This inhibition causes muscle relaxation and consequently results in further ROM increase.[115]

This proposed mode of action contains an erroneous premise. Under normal circumstances, when a person is fully relaxed there is no motor tone in the muscles, i.e. there is no demonstrable activity on the EMG trace.[117–120] Similarly, when a person is stretched passively the muscle is motorically silent. If muscle activity is observed, it is usually when the stretching reaches the end-range of movement at the onset of discomfort and pain (Fig. 8.9).[99,100,121] This increase in motor activity is likely to be an evasive response to pain. It means that during the early phase of stretching the muscle is relaxed and therefore further inhibition is not possible – *cannot relax a relaxed muscle* – whereas, at the end-ranges, motor activity is likely to increase; an outcome which would defeat this particular treatment goal (muscle relaxation).

Another way to look at inhibition is to examine the gain of the spinal motoneurons. A high gain would suggest that the muscle is close to the threshold of being activated, whereas reduced gain implies central relaxation and reduced potential for activation. There are several studies that demonstrate a (very) transient gain attenuation of spinal motor centres during passive stretching.[115,122–124] However, these influences are unlikely to be physiologically or therapeutically significant. This is because the gain of spinal motor centres is

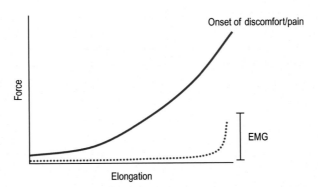

FIGURE 8.9 During passive stretching the muscle is motorically silent. Electromyography (EMG) activity may be observed when stretching begins to be uncomfortable or painful.

heavily modulated by descending signals from higher motor centres, but only minimally by the reflexive influences from mechanoreceptors.[125] The dominance of the central process over peripheral stimulation has important implications for passive stretching. It means that the individual's intention to consciously relax the muscle will have a far more dominant inhibitory effect on spinal motoneurons than the peripherally induced inhibition. It is also more likely to outlast any reflexive stimulation.[116] A simple verbal, cognitive instruction to the patient to relax their muscle ("make the areas soft") may be far more beneficial than numerous repeated stretches.

Furthermore, spinal motoneurons are continuously varying their gain according to the background task (*task-dependent reflexes*) and not by peripheral mechanisms which serve to provide feedback.[22,23,126,127] For example, when the cutaneous afferents of the paw of a walking cat are stimulated during the swing phase (as the limb is moving into flexion) it reinforces the flexion movement. When the same stimulus is applied during leg extension it reinforces extension.[128] Similarly, the gain of the stretch reflex is modulated during the human walking cycle.[129] The amplitude of the quadriceps stretch reflex is increased while the limb is moving into extension but inhibited when the limb is moving into flexion. Even when the human cutaneous afferents in the leg are stimulated it results in inhibitory or excitatory motor responses depending on the current posture or activity.[130]

Another persistent misconception is that techniques such as METs can result in autogenic inhibition. This inhibition is believed to occur by stimulation of the Golgi tendon organ (GTO) during contraction.[115,116] These receptors are sensitive to muscle contraction and, indeed, in laboratory studies stimulation of GTOs has been shown to have a weak inhibitory influence on the spinal motoneurons (often when central or descending influences from higher centres are eliminated).[131–133] However, in "real life" the descending influences override the peripherally mediated inhibition; if it were any different, humans would have reached an evolutionary dead-end long ago. Just imagine hanging over the side of a cliff. The muscle tendon units are now on maximum tension and the GTOs are fully excited. Under these circumstances there is full reflex inhibition from the GTOs. According to the autogenic inhibition assumption, the arm muscles should be relaxing, a response which would be extremely disadvantageous in this situation. Fortunately this scenario does not happen. The dominance of central motor centres overrides these mild peripheral influences.

What about post-contraction inhibition? Yes, it can be demonstrated in laboratory studies, but it is a very weak, transient response that occurs in milliseconds. It is completely overrun by the motor requirements of the successive task (see task-dependent reflexes above). Just imagine what would happen to the ensuing activity if inhibition was present every time we contracted a muscle – we would never be able to perform the next task as we would be in a state of inhibition sustained from the previous task.

Overall, there is no support in the science (or more importantly logic) for autogenic inhibition as a mechanism for elongation in passive stretching or METs.[116]

Reciprocal inhibition

There is another widespread belief in manual therapy that, during METs, the isometric contraction of agonists will reciprocally inhibit the antagonistic muscles. However, there are several factors which call into question the therapeutic value of reciprocal inhibition.

Reciprocal inhibition occurs when the tendon of an actively contracting muscle is tapped. It results in an observable drop in the antagonist muscle's EMG amplitude and contraction force. This response is weak, non-functional and lasts only a few milliseconds; it cannot be induced continuously (tonically).[134,135] Furthermore, reciprocal inhibition is a research phenomenon, a physiological artefact observable during laboratory studies.[131] However, it does not occur during normal movement. Under normal circumstances, the control to synergistic pairs is simultaneous and centrally controlled (Fig. 8.10).[1] It is not controlled from the periphery by stimulation of mechanoreceptors.[41]

Furthermore, during movement there is often co-contraction of synergistic pairs, which means no reciprocal inhibition (Box 8.1). Such co-contraction has been demonstrated during the active phase of METs/PNF.[98,136,137] In a study of METs, we were able to demonstrate that concurrent triceps co-contract during biceps METs. The greater the force of biceps contraction, the greater

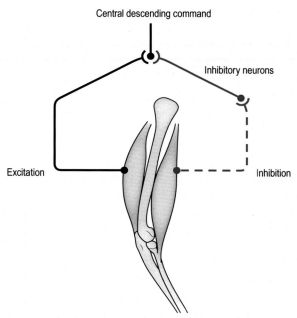

FIGURE 8.10 Inhibition and excitation of the synergistic muscles by central command occurs simultaneously. It is not controlled from the periphery by mechanoreceptors.

the co-contraction in the triceps (Fig. 8.11).[138] If reciprocal inhibition were present, we should not have seen any EMG activity in the triceps muscle during biceps contraction.

Overall, manual techniques, active or passive, that rely on proprioceptive reflexes are unlikely to have any significant effect on movement control or play any significant role in active ROM recovery (see summary in Box 8.2).[41]

SUMMARY

- The organization of movement is whole and integrated with its goals
- The use of an external focus of attention and goal-orientated movement strategies is more beneficial for control and recovery of movement
- Internal focusing strategies on specific muscles or joints turns them into the goal of movement and reduces the effectiveness of rehabilitation
- Regression to internal focus may be necessary in situations when task performance is not possible
- Muscle activity is task dependent: muscle recruitment sequences are unique to each task; training-specific control of muscles in one task may fail to improve the control of a different task

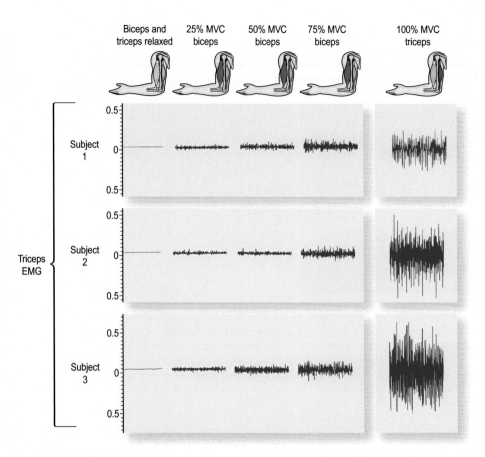

FIGURE 8.11 Co-contraction of triceps during specific isometric biceps contraction in three subjects. As the force of biceps contraction increases, at 25%, 50% and 75% maximal voluntary contraction (MVC), there is a concurrent increase in triceps electromyography (EMG) activity. For comparison in the right column: EMG of triceps during 100% MVC. Co-contraction of triceps was present in all 30 subjects who participated in this study. *Reprinted from Lederman E. The Science and Practice of Manual Therapy, 2005, with permission from Elsevier.*

- There are four task parameters that can be challenged during ROM rehabilitation: force, velocity, range/angle and endurance
- The task parameters should be challenged within-task and not targeted as individual muscles or muscle chains
- Regression to focusing on single muscles, muscle chains or specific joints should be the last option in any treatment
- Active ROM should be rehabilitated with active movement (Table 8.1)
- ROM rehabilitation should be of whole movement, goal orientated and within the context of functional tasks (Table 8.1)
- *Think control not individual muscles*

Table 8.1 The potential of different range of movement (ROM) challenges to help recover motor control

	Management/ROM challenge	Active?	Goal and whole?	
Functional	Recovery behaviour	Yes	Yes	Most effective for active ROM
	Managed recovery behaviour	Yes	Yes	
	Assisted recovery behaviour (functional stretching)	Yes	Yes	
Extra-functional	Ballistic stretching	Yes	No	
	Dynamic stretching	Yes	No (not often)	
	Muscle energy techniques	Yes	No	
	Passive stretching	No	No	
	Spinal manipulation	No	No	
	Traction	No	No	
	Articulation	No	No	
	Harmonic	No	No	
	Strain counter-strain	No	No	
	Cranial	No	No	Least effective

BOX 8.1 FEEL THE SYNERGY

There are two principal synergistic patterns that can be experienced by a simple exercise. While standing, draw large imaginary numbers, 0 to 10, with your arm in space; then repeat the same exercise, but now draw smaller numbers fast. You will notice that when drawing fast, small numbers the muscles around the shoulder and the trunk tend to stiffen. This pattern of recruitment is called co-contraction. This is different from the on–off, *reciprocal–activation* pattern experienced during the slow, large number drawing. Co-contraction is the simultaneous activation of several muscle groups to stabilize joints during static postures (static stabilization or steadiness) or to stabilize during movement (dynamic stabilization). Co-contraction also has a role in refining movement, which is why it is felt during fast, small-amplitude movement. Reciprocal activation is often associated with the control of dynamic movement.[22,23,139–143]

BOX 8.2

Key points on passive and reflexive approaches

Manual techniques or exercise that relies on reflex mechanisms to improve range of movement are likely to be ineffective on several grounds:

1. The role of proprioceptors is to provide feedback; they are not control systems. Inhibition and excitation are their modes of communication.[42]
2. Higher centres dominate spinal motor centres and can modify or override the weaker proprioceptive influences.
3. The influence of proprioceptors on spinal motor gain is very transient. This gain would be reset completely by the control demands of any ensuing movement. This could even be in advance of the movement: spinal motor centres are recruited in anticipation of movement, even before proprioceptive feedback becomes available from the movement.[68]

Passive stretching approaches are in conflict with several of the motor control principles:

1. Motor learning and functional movement is active. Motor control cannot be recovered by passive challenges (e.g. spinal manipulation). During passive techniques there is no active motor engagement.
2. Task-specific recruitment is not being practised.
3. There is an absence of movement goals.
4. Passive stretching represents a profoundly fragmented approach that reduces the movement to the level of the muscle and the (ineffective) reflexive.

REFERENCES

1. Hughlings-Jackson J. On the comparative study of disease of the nervous system. Br Med J 1889;17:355–62.
2. Hommel B, Prinz W. Toward an action-concept model of stimulus–response compatibility. In: Hommel B, Prinz W, editors. Theoretical issues in stimulus–response compatibility. Amsterdam: Elsevier; 1997.
3. Rosenbaum DA, Meulenbroek RGJ, Vaughan J. What is the point of motor planning? Int J Sport Exerc Psychol 2004;2:439–69.
4. Koch I, Keller R, Prinz W. The ideomotor approach to action control: implication for skilled performance. Int J Sport Exerc Psychol 2004;2:362–75.
5. Elsner B, Hommel B. Effect anticipation and action control. J Exp Psychol Hum Percept Perform 2001;27(1):229–40.
6. Shadmehr R. Generalization as a behavioral window to the neural mechanisms of learning internal models. Hum Move Sci 2004;23:543–68.
7. Reeves NP, Everding VQ, Cholewicki J, et al. The effects of trunk stiffness on postural control during unstable seated balance. Exp Brain Res 2006;174(4):694–700.
8. McNevin NH, Wulf G, Carlson C. Effects of attentional focus, self-control, and dyad training on motor learning: implications for physical rehabilitation. Phys Ther 2000;80(4):373–85.
9. McNevin NH, Shea CH, Wulf G. Increasing the distance of an external focus of attention enhances learning. Psychol Res 2003;67(1):22–9.
10. Wulf G, McConnel N, Gärtner M, et al. Enhancing the learning of sport skills through external-focus feedback. J Mot Behav 2002;34(2):171–82.
11. Wulf G, Weigelt M, Poulter D, et al. Attentional focus on suprapostural tasks affects balance learning. Q J Exp Psychol A 2003;56(7):1191–211.
12. Beilock SL, Carr TH, MacMahon C, et al. When paying attention becomes counterproductive: impact of divided versus skill-focused attention on novice and experienced performance of sensorimotor skills. J Exp Psychol Appl 2002;8(1):6–16.
13. Kurtzer I, DiZio P, Lackner J. Task-dependent motor learning. Exp Brain Res 2003;153(1):128–32.
14. Zachry T, Wulf G, Mercer J, et al. Increased movement accuracy and reduced EMG activity as the result of adopting an external focus of attention. Brain Res Bull 2005;67(4):304–9.
15. Vance J, Wulf G, Töllner T, et al. EMG activity as a function of the performer's focus of attention. J Mot Behav 2004;36(4):450–9.
16. Marchant D, Greig M, Scott C. Attentional focusing instructions influence force production and muscular activity during isokinetic elbow flexions. J Strength Condit Res 2009;23:2358–66.
17. Lohse KR, Sherwood DE, Healy AF. Neuromuscular effects of shifting the focus of attention in a simple force production task. J Mot Behav 2011;43(2):173–84.
18. Wulf G, Dufek JS, Lozano L, et al. Increased jump height and reduced EMG activity with an external focus. Hum Mov Sci 2010;29(3):440–8.
19. Wulf G, Dufek JS. Increased jump height with an external focus due to enhanced lower extremity joint kinetics. J Mot Behav 2009;41(5):401–9.
20. Brown SH, Vera-Garcia FJ, McGill SM. Effects of abdominal muscle coactivation on the externally preloaded trunk: variations in motor control and its effect on spine stability. Spine 2006;31(13):E387–93.
21. Totsika V, Wulf G. The influence of external and internal foci of attention on transfer to novel situations and skills. Res Q Exerc Sport 2003;74(2):220–5.
22. Doemges F, Rack P. Changes in the stretch reflex of the human first interosseous muscle during different tasks. J Physiol 1992;447:563–73.
23. Doemges F, Rack P. Task-dependent changes in the response of human wrist joints to mechanical disturbance. J Physiol 1992;447:575–85.

24. Hore J, McCloskey DI, Taylor JL. Task-dependent changes in gain of the reflex response to imperceptible perturbations of joint position in man. J Physiol 1990;429:309–21.
25. Weiss EJ, Flanders M. Muscular and postural synergies of the human hand. J Neurophysiol 2004;92(1):523–35.
26. McGill SM, Grenier S, Kavcic N, et al. Coordination of muscle activity to assure stability of the lumbar spine. J Electromyogr Kinesiol 2003;13(4):353–9.
27. Carpenter MG, Tokuno CD, Thorstensson A, et al. Differential control of abdominal muscles during multi-directional support-surface translations in man. Exp Brain Res 2008;188(3): 445–55.
28. Kavcic N, Grenier S, McGill SM. Determining the stabilizing role of individual torso muscles during rehabilitation exercises. Spine 2004;29(11):1254–65.
29. Andersson EA, Oddsson LI, Grundstrom H, et al. EMG activities of the quadratus lumborum and erector spinae muscles during flexion-relaxation and other motor tasks. Clin Biomech 1996;11:392–400.
30. Urquhart DM, Hodges PW, Story IH. Postural activity of the abdominal muscles varies between regions of these muscles and between body positions. Gait Posture 2005;22(4): 295–301.
31. Leirdal S, Roeleveld K, Ettema G. Coordination specificity in strength and power training. Int J Sports Med 2008;29(3):225–31.
32. Young WB, Rath DA. Enhancing foot velocity in football kicking: the role of strength training. J Strength Cond Res 2011;25(2):561–6.
33. Godges JJ, MacRae PG, Engelke KA. Effects of exercise on hip range of motion, trunk muscle performance, and gait economy. Phys Ther 1993;73(7):468–77.
34. Bjørn A, Hoff J. Coordination, the determinant of velocity specificity? J Appl Physiol 1996;80(5):2046–52.
35. Weir JP, Keefe DA, Eaton JF, et al. Effect of fatigue on hamstring coactivation during isokinetic knee extensions. Eur J Appl Physiol Occup Physiol 1998;78(6):555–9.
36. Maynard J, Ebben WP. The effects of antagonist prefatigue on agonist torque and electromyography. J Strength Cond Res 2003;17(3):469–74.
37. Semmler JG, Tucker KJ, Allen TJ, et al. Eccentric exercise increases EMG amplitude and force fluctuations during submaximal contractions of elbow flexor muscles. J Appl Physiol 2007;103(3):979–89.
38. Nyland JA, Caborn DN, Shapiro R. Fatigue after eccentric quadriceps femoris work produces earlier gastrocnemius and delayed quadriceps femoris activation during crossover cutting among normal athletic women. Knee Surg Sports Traumatol Arthrosc 1997;5(3): 162–7.
39. Thomas JS, France CR, Sha D, et al. The effect of chronic low back pain on trunk muscle activations in target reaching movements with various loads. Spine 2007;32(26):E801–8.
40. Thomas JS, France CR, Lavender SA, et al. Effects of fear of movement on spine velocity and acceleration after recovery from low back pain. Spine 2008;33(5):564–70.
41. Lederman E. The science and practice of manual therapy. Edinburgh: Elsevier; 2005.
42. Lederman E. Neuromuscular rehabilitation in manual and physical therapies. Edinburgh: Elsevier; 2010.
43. Jones DW, Jones DA, Newham DJ. Chronic knee effusion and aspiration: the effect on quadriceps inhibition. Br J Rheumatol 1987;26:370–4.
44. Stokes M, Young A. The contribution of reflex inhibition to arthrogenous muscle weakness. Clin Sci 1984;67:7–14.
45. Stokes JF, Stokes M, Young A. Reflex actions of knee joint afferents during contraction of the human quadriceps. Clin Physiol 1990;10:489–500.
46. Spencer JD, Hayes KC, Alexander IJ. Knee joint effusion and quadriceps reflex inhibition in man. Arch Phys Med Rehabil 1984;65:171–7.
47. Hurley MV, O'Flanagan SJ, Newham DJ. Isokinetic and isometric muscle strength and inhibition after elbow arthroplasty. J Orthop Rheumatol 1991;4:83–95.

48. Hides JA, Stokes MJ, Saide M, et al. Evidence of lumbar multifidus muscle wasting ipsilateral to symptoms in patients with acute/subacute low back pain. Spine 1994;19(2):165–72.

49. Raghavan P, Krakauer JW, Gordon AM. Impaired anticipatory control of fingertip forces in patients with a pure motor or sensorimotor lacunar syndrome. Brain 2006;129(Pt 6):1415–25.

50. Fellows SJ, Noth J, Schwarz M. Precision grip and Parkinson's disease. Brain 1998;121 (Pt 9):1771–84.

51. Shirado O, Ito T, Kaneda K, Strax TE. Concentric and eccentric strength of trunk muscles: influence of test postures on strength and characteristics of patients with chronic low-back pain. Arch Phys Med Rehabil 1995;76(7):604–11.

52. Shirado O, Ito T, Kaneda K, et al. Flexion–relaxation phenomenon in the back muscles: a comparative study between healthy subjects and patients with chronic low back pain. Am J Phys Med Rehabil 1995;74(2):139–44.

53. Lamoth CJ, Meijer OG, Daffertshofer A, et al. Effects of chronic low back pain on trunk coordination and back muscle activity during walking: changes in motor control. Eur Spine J 2006;15(1):23–40.

54. Lamoth CJ, Daffertshofer A, Meijer OG, et al. How do persons with chronic low back pain speed up and slow down? Trunk–pelvis coordination and lumbar erector spinae activity during gait. Gait Posture 2006;23(2):230–9.

55. Thomas JS, France CR, Lavender SA, et al. Effects of fear of movement on spine velocity and acceleration after recovery from low back pain. Spine 2008;33(5):564–70.

56. Zedka M, Prochazka A, Knight B, et al. Voluntary and reflex control of human back muscles during induced pain. J Physiol 1999;520(Pt 2):591–604.

57. Bandholm T, Rasmussen L, Aagaard P, et al. Force steadiness, muscle activity, and maximal muscle strength in subjects with subacromial impingement syndrome. Muscle Nerve 2006; 34(5):631–9.

58. Bandholm T, Rasmussen L, Aagaard P, et al. Effects of experimental muscle pain on shoulder-abduction force steadiness and muscle activity in healthy subjects. Eur J Appl Physiol 2008;102(6):643–50.

59. Kumbhare DA. Measurement of cervical flexor endurance following whiplash. Disabil Rehabil 2005;27(14):801–7.

60. Suter E, Lindsay D. Back muscle fatigability is associated with knee extensor inhibition in subjects with low back pain. Spine 2001;26(16):E361–6.

61. Roy SH, De Luca CJ, Casavant DA. Lumbar muscle fatigue and chronic lower back pain. Spine 1989;14(9):992–1001.

62. Smits-Engelsman BC, Rameckers EA, Duysens J. Muscle force generation and force control of finger movements in children with spastic hemiplegia during isometric tasks. Dev Med Child Neurol 2005;47(5):337–42.

63. Rameckers EA, Smits-Engelsman BC, Duysens J. Children with spastic hemiplegia are equally able as controls in maintaining a precise percentage of maximum force without visually monitoring their performance. Neuropsychologia 2005;43(13):1938–45.

64. Prodoehl J, MacKinnon CD, Comella CL, et al. Strength deficits in primary focal hand dystonia. Mov Disord 2006;21(1):18–27.

65. Yazawa S, Ikeda A, Kaji R, et al. Abnormal cortical processing of voluntary muscle relaxation in patients with focal hand dystonia studied by movement-related potentials. Brain 1999;122(Pt 7):1357–66.

66. Fitts PM, Posner MI. Human performance. London: Brooks/Cole; 1967.

67. Magill RA. Motor learning concepts and applications. Dubuque, IA: William C Brown; 1985.

68. Schmidt RA, Lee TD. Motor control and learning. 4th edn. Champaign, IL: Human Kinetics; 2005.

69. McEwen SE, Huijbregts MP, Ryan JD, et al. Cognitive strategy use to enhance motor skill acquisition post-stroke: a critical review. Brain Inj 2009;23(4):263–77.

70. McEwen SE, Polatajko HJ, Huijbregts MP, et al. Inter-task transfer of meaningful, functional skills following a cognitive-based treatment: results of three multiple baseline design experiments in adults with chronic stroke. Neuropsychol Rehabil 2010;20(4):541–61.
71. Judd CH. The relation of special training to general intelligence. Educ Rev 1908;36:28–42.
72. Arthur JC, Philbeck JW, Chichka D. Non-sensory inputs to angular path integration. J Vestib Res 2009;19(3–4):111–25.
73. Levack WM, Taylor K, Siegert RJ, et al. Is goal planning in rehabilitation effective? A systematic review. Clin Rehabil 2006;20(9):739–55.
74. Sivaraman Nair KP. Life goals: the concept and its relevance to rehabilitation. Clin Rehabil 2003;17(2):192–202.
75. Soberg HL, Finset A, Roise O, et al. Identification and comparison of rehabilitation goals after multiple injuries: an ICF analysis of the patients', physiotherapists' and other allied professionals' reported goals. J Rehabil Med 2008;40(5):340–6.
76. Chan DK, Lonsdale C, Ho PY, et al. Patient motivation and adherence to postsurgery rehabilitation exercise recommendations: the influence of physiotherapists' autonomy-supportive behaviors. Arch Phys Med Rehabil 2009;90(12):1977–82.
77. Saxton JM, Clarkson PM, James R, et al. Neuromuscular dysfunction following eccentric exercise. Med Sci Sports Exerc 1995;27(8):1185–93.
78. Bonfim TR, Jansen Paccola CA, Barela JA. Proprioceptive and behavior impairments in individuals with anterior cruciate ligament reconstructed knees. Arch Phys Med Rehabil 2003;84:1217–23.
79. Lackner R, DiZio P. Adaptation to Coriolis force perturbation of movement trajectory: role of proprioceptive and cutaneous somatosensory feedback. Adv Exp Med Biol 2002;508:69–78.
80. Bobath B. The application of physiological principles to stroke rehabilitation. Practitioner 1979;223:793–4.
81. Held R. Plasticity in sensorimotor coordination. In: Freedman SJ, editor. The neuropsychology of spatially oriented behavior. Homewood, IL: Dorsey Press; 1968.
82. Taub E. Movement in nonhuman primates deprived of somatosensory feedback. Exerc Sports Sci Rev 4:335–74.
83. Taub E, Berman A. Movement and learning in the absence of sensory feedback. In: Freedman SJ, editor. The neurophysiology of spatially orientated behavior. Homewood, IL: Dorsey Press; 1968.
84. Blennerhassett J, Dite W. Additional task-related practice improves mobility and upper limb function early after stroke: a randomised controlled trial. Aust J Physiother 2004;50:219–24.
85. Carey LM, Matyas TA. Frequency of discriminative sensory loss in the hand after stroke in a rehabilitation setting. J Rehabil Med 2011;43(3):257–63.
86. Holding DH. Principles of training. London: Pergamon Press; 1965.
87. Gardner EP. Somatosensory cortical mechanisms of feature detection in tactile and kinesthetic discrimination. Can J Physiol Pharmacol 1987;66:439–54.
88. Roland PE. Sensory feedback to the cerebral cortex during voluntary movement in man. Behav Brain Sci 1978;1:129–71.
89. Lemon RN, Porter R. Short-latency peripheral afferent inputs to pyramidal and other neurones in the precentral cortex of conscious monkeys. In: Gordon G, editor. Active touch. Oxford: Pergamon Press; 1978:91–103.
90. Elliott D, Grierson LE, Hayes SJ, et al. Action representations in perception, motor control and learning: implications for medical education. Med Educ 2011;45(2):119–31.
91. Maxwell JP, Masters RS, Eves FF. From novice to no know-how: a longitudinal study of implicit motor learning. J Sports Sci 2000;18(2):111–20.
92. Dickinson J. The training of mobile balancing under a minimal visual cue situation. Ergonomics 1966;11:169–75.

93. Winstein CJ, Pohl PS, Lewthwaite R. Effects of physical guidance and knowledge of results on motor learning: support for the guidance hypothesis. Res Q Exerc Sport 1994;65(4): 316–23.

94. Weeks DL, Kordus RN. Relative frequency of knowledge of performance and motor skill learning. Res Q Exerc Sport 1998;69(3):224–30.

95. Schmidt RA, Wulf G. Continuous concurrent feedback degrades skill learning: implications for training and simulation. Hum Factors 1997;39(4):509–25.

96. Chiviacowsky S, Wulf G. Feedback after good trials enhances learning. Res Q Exerc Sport 2007;78(2):40–7.

97. Shellock FG, Prentice WE. Warming-up and stretching for improved physical performance and prevention of sports-related injuries. Sports Med 1985;2(4):267–78.

98. Magnusson SP, Aagard P, Simonsen E, et al. A biomechanical evaluation of cyclic and static stretch in human skeletal muscle. Int J Sports Med 1998;19:310–16.

99. Klinge K, Magnusson SP, Simonsen EB, et al. The effect of strength and flexibility training on skeletal muscle electromyographic activity, stiffness and viscoelastic stress relaxation response. Am J Sports Med 1997;25(5):710–16.

100. Halbertsma JP, Göeken LN, Hof AL, et al. Extensibility and stiffness of the hamstrings in patients with nonspecific low back pain. Arch Phys Med Rehabil 2001;82(2):232–8.

101. Dockery ML, Wright TW, LaStayo PC. Electromyography of the shoulder: an analysis of passive modes of exercise. Orthopedics 1998;21(11):1181–4.

102. Newham DJ, Lederman E. Effect of manual therapy techniques on the stretch reflex in normal human quadriceps. Disabil Rehabil 1997;19(8):326–31.

103. Klam F, Graf W. Discrimination between active and passive head movements by macaque ventral and medial intraparietal cortex neurons. J Physiol 2006;574(Pt 2):367–86.

104. Ciccarelli O, Toosy AT, Marsden JF, et al. Identifying brain regions for integrative sensori-motor processing with ankle movements. Exp Brain Res 2005;166(1):31–42.

105. Mima T, Sadato N, Yazawa S, et al. Brain structures related to active and passive finger movements in man. Brain 1999;122(10):1989–97.

106. Sahyoun C, Floyer-Lea A, Johansen-Berg H, et al. Towards an understanding of gait control: brain activation during the anticipation, preparation and execution of foot movements. Neuroimage 2004;21(2):568–75.

107. Obhi SS, Planetta PJ, Scantlebury J. On the signals underlying conscious awareness of action. Cognition 2009;110(1):65–73.

108. Shadmehr R, Maurice A, Smith MA, et al. Error correction, sensory prediction, and adaptation in motor control. Annu Rev Neurosci 2010;33:89–108.

109. Lloyd AJ, Caldwell LS. Accuracy of active and passive positioning of the leg on the basis of kinesthetic cues. J Comp Physiol Psychol 1965 60(1):102–6.

110. Paillard J, Brouchon M. Active and passive movements in the calibration of position sense. In: Freedman SJ, editor. The neuropsychology of spatially oriented behavior. Homewood, IL: Dorsey Press; 1968:37–55.

111. Féry YA, Magnac R, Israël I. Commanding the direction of passive whole-body rotations facilitates egocentric spatial updating. Cognition 2004;91(2):B1–10.

112. Gandevia SC, McCloskey DI. Joint sense, muscle sense and their combination as position sense, measured at the distal interphalangeal joint of the middle finger. J Physiol 1976;260: 387–407.

113. Silfies SP, Cholewicki J, Reeves NP, Greene HS. Lumbar position sense and the risk of low back injuries in college athletes: a prospective cohort study. BMC Musculoskelet Disord 2007;8:129.

114. Weiller C, Jüptner M, Fellows S, et al. Brain representation of active and passive movements. Neuroimage 1996;4(2):105–10.

115. Etnyre BR, Abraham LD. H-reflex changes during static stretching and two variations of proprioceptive neuromuscular facilitation techniques. Electroencephalogr Clin Neurophysiol 1986;63(2):174–9.

116. Chalmers G. Re-examination of the possible role of Golgi tendon organ and muscle spindle reflexes in proprioceptive neuromuscular facilitation muscle stretching. Sports Biomech 2004;3(1):159–83.

117. Clemmesen S. Some studies of muscle tone. Proc R Soc Med 1951;44:637–46.

118. Basmajian JV. New views on muscular tone and relaxation. Can Med Assoc J 1957;77: 203–5.

119. Basmajian JV. Muscles alive: their function revealed by electromyography. Baltimore, MD: Williams & Wilkins; 1978.

120. Ralston HJ, Libet B. The question of tonus in skeletal muscles. Am J Phys Med 1953;32:85–92.

121. Magnusson SP, Simonsen EB, Aagaard P, et al. Determinants of musculoskeletal flexibility: viscoelastic properties, cross-sectional area, EMG and stretch tolerance. Scand J Med Sci Sports 1997;7:195–202.

122. Guissard N, Duchateau J, Hainaut K. Muscle stretching and motoneuron excitability. Eur J Appl Physiol Occup Physiol 1988;58(1–2):47–52.

123. Guissard N, Duchateau J, Hainaut K. Mechanisms of decreased motoneurone excitation during passive muscle stretching. Exp Brain Res 2001;137(2):163–9.

124. Guissard N, Duchateau J. Neural aspects of muscle stretching. Exerc Sport Sci Rev 2006;34(4):154–8.

125. Bennett DJ, Gorassini M, Prochazka A. Catching a ball: contribution of intrinsic muscle stiffness, reflexes, and higher order responses. Can J Physiol Pharmacol 1994;72(2): 525–34.

126. Evarts EV. Brain mechanisms in voluntary movement. In: Mcfadden D, editor. Neural mechanisms in behavior. New York: Springer; 1980.

127. Gielen C, Ramaekers L, van Zuylen E. Long latency stretch reflexes as co-ordinated functional responses in man. J Physiol 1988;407:275–92.

128. Forssberg H, Grillner S, Rossignol S. Phase dependent reflex reversal during walking in chronic spinal cat. Brain Res 1975;85:103–7.

129. Capaday C, Stein RB. Difference in the amplitude of the human soleus H-reflex during walking and running. J Physiol 392:513–22.

130. Burke D, Dickson HG, Skuse NF. Task dependent changes in the responses to low-threshold cutaneous afferent volleys in the human lower limb. J Physiol 1991;432: 445–58.

131. Matthews PBC. Muscle spindles: their messages and their fusimotor supply. In: Brookhart JM, Mountcastle VB, Brooks VB, editors. Motor control, Pt 1, Handbook of physiology, Sect 1, vol 2. Bethesda, MD: American Physiological Society; 1981:189–228.

132. Jami L. Golgi tendon organs in mammalian skeletal muscle: functional properties and central actions. Physiol Rev 1992;73(3):623–66.

133. Gregory JE, Brockett CL, Morgan DL, et al. Effect of eccentric muscle contractions on Golgi tendon organ responses to passive and active tension in the cat. J Physiol 2002;1;538 (Pt 1):209–18.

134. Cody FWJ, Plant T. Vibration-evoked reciprocal inhibition between human wrist muscles. Brain Res 1989;78:613–23.

135. Belanger AY, Morin S, Pepin P, et al. Manual muscle tapping decreases soleus H-reflex amplitude in control subjects. Physiother Can 1989;41(4):192–6.

136. Osternig LR, Robertson R, Troxel R, et al. Muscle activation during proprioceptive neuromuscular facilitation (PNF) stretching techniques. Am J Phys Med 1987;66(5): 298–307.

137. Mitchell UH, Myrer JW, Hopkins JT, et al. Neurophysiological reflex mechanisms' lack of contribution to the success of PNF stretches. J Sport Rehabil 2009;18(3):343–57.

138. Lederman E, Vaz M. Co-contraction of triceps during isometric activity in biceps brachii: implications to muscle energy technique. ICAOR conference, London (abstract available at www.cpdo.net).

139. Labriola JE, Lee TQ, Debski RE, et al. Stability and instability of the glenohumeral joint: the role of shoulder muscles. J Shoulder Elbow Surg 2005;14(1 Suppl S):32S–8S.
140. Yanagawa T, Goodwin CJ, Shelburne KB, et al. Contributions of the individual muscles of the shoulder to glenohumeral joint stability during abduction. J Biomech Eng 2008; 130(2):021024.
141. Gribble PL, Mullin LI, Cothros N, et al. Role of cocontraction in arm movement accuracy. J Neurophysiol 2003;89(5):2396–405.
142. Granata KP, Marras WS. Cost–benefit of muscle cocontraction in protecting against spinal instability. Spine 2000;25(11):1398–404.
143. van Dieen JH, Kingma I, van der Bug JCE. Evidence for a role of antagonistic cocontraction in controlling trunk stiffness during lifting. J Biomech 2003;36:1829–36.

CHAPTER 9

Pain Management and ROM Desensitization

Imagine three clinical scenarios in which patients present with different knee conditions. The first patient presents with a knee sprain which happened 1 week ago. It is painful, swollen and stiff and on examination has only a limited range of movement (ROM). Another patient had a knee joint fracture. It is now 6 weeks later and the plaster has just been removed. The knee is painful, swollen, has restricted ROM and is very stiff. Finally, another patient had knee surgery 1 year ago. On examination the passive knee ranges have mostly recovered but pain and stiffness are still limiting the patient's functional ranges.

The clinical examples above represent three conditions in which pain, stiffness and ROM losses are shared symptoms. However, the ROM management will be different for each of these presentations. These scenarios raise several questions about ROM rehabilitation in the presence of pain:

- In the presence of pain, when is stretching/ROM challenge safe or useful?
- When is pain a signal to stop stretching?
- How soon after injury should ROM challenges commence?
- Can movement be stiff and painful without inflammation, damage or shortening?
- What is ROM sensitization?
- What can help to promote desensitization?
- Can stretching be used to control pain?

ROM SENSITIZATION

Sensitization is a neurological process in which the central nervous system can change, distort or amplify the experience of pain in a manner that no longer reflects the noxious stimuli from the periphery.[1] ROM sensitization is the limitation in ROM owing to an increase in the subjective experience of stiffness and pain. It is a common phenomenon in acute and chronic musculoskeletal conditions.[2] Of particular focus here is ROM sensitization in which pain and

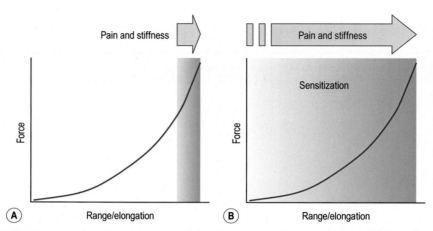

FIGURE 9.1 Range of movement (ROM) sensitization. A. Under normal circumstances pain and stiffness are experienced at end-ranges. B. In the presence of sensitization, pain and stiffness are experience within normal non-noxious ROM and as severe pain at end-ranges.

stiffness are experienced in functional ranges, in the absence of current tissue damage, inflammation or tissue shortening (Fig. 9.1). This phenomenon will be termed here *persistent ROM sensitization*.

Under normal circumstances sensitization is a *positive* protective response to injury. Following injury, the site of damage, as well as its surrounding area, will become hypersensitive to touch, movement or temperature. This sensitivity serves as a warning system to protect the weakened tissues from further damage.[3]

Sensitization is brought about by increased excitability of nociceptors in the periphery and central neurons that convey the nociceptive information. Peripherally, inflammatory by-products lower the nociceptors' threshold, resulting in their increased excitability.[4-8] Centrally, within the spinal cord and brain, sensitization is associated with complex biological and functional reorganization of sensory transmission and motor and autonomic responses. The outcome is facilitation and amplification of nociceptive signals throughout the nervous system.[9-16]

Sensitization tends to spread in the spinal cord to influence the receptive field of neurons that are not directly related to the site of injury. This spread can even affect the receptive fields of spinal neurons on the non-affected side.[7,8] This means that pain sensitivity can be experienced further away from the site of injury as well as on the opposite limb. For example, in some patients with osteoarthritis of the hip there is increased pain perception and skin sensitivity at locations distant to the joint and even on the non-affected side.[17]

The consequence of sensitization is an elevated pain experience which is disproportionate to underlying tissue strain or damage (Fig. 9.2). Such hypersensitivity means that previously normal functional ranges are experienced as painful, and end-ranges which were uncomfortable become intolerably painful.

Persistent sensitization

Under normal circumstances pain and sensitization tend to diminish as the individual recovers from their injury. However, for some individuals persistent central sensitization can be maintained long after tissue healing has taken place (Fig. 9.3). It can arise spontaneously, even without an obvious event of injury. Once central sensitization has taken place it does not seem to be dependent any longer on nociception from the damaged tissues.[11] Indeed, in many chronic pain conditions there is an absence of "fresh" tissue damage or inflammation.[1,18] Consequently, *persistent sensitization may lead the patient (and the therapist) to the erroneous belief that the painful area is damaged and inflamed.*

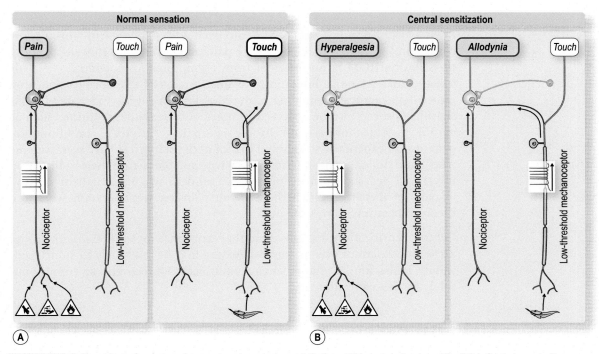

FIGURE 9.2 Neural mechanisms of normal and central sensizitation. *With permission from Woolf CJ. Central sensization: implications for the diagnosis and treatment of pain. Pain 2011;152(3 suppl):S2–15. These figures have been reproduced with permission of the International Association for the Study of Pain ® (IASP). The figures may NOT be reproduced for any other purpose without permission.*

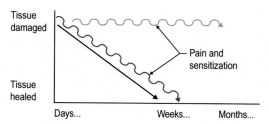

FIGURE 9.3 The experience of pain and sensitization tends to diminish in line with tissue healing. In some situations it can persist in the absence of tissue damage.

Persistent pain sensitization is a feature of many chronic musculoskeletal conditions.[1] It can be demonstrated in injury/post-surgical conditions,[19] chronic low back and neck pain, trapezius myalgia, whiplash conditions, painful jaw and post-immobilization.[1,20-25] Sensitization also plays a role in the various tendinopathies such as tennis elbow and supraspinatous, Achilles and patellar tendinopathies.[26-31] In arthritis, both joint nociceptors and related spinal nociceptive neurons show pronounced sensitization for mechanical stimulation.[32]

ROM sensitization has also been demonstrated in patients with chronic low back pain.[33] Athough they experience pain and stiffness in forward bending their flexion ROM is no different from asymptomatic individuals.[34-37] This suggests that the range limitation was due to reduced tolerance to stretching rather than physical shortening of the muscles.[33] A similar example of ROM sensitization can also be observed in non-traumatic pain conditions such as chronic trapezius myalgia and chronic neck pain.[22-25] In these conditions, the patient may experience substantial loss of neck rotation. (I have seen patients who could no longer drive because they were unable to turn their head during reversing.) Yet, such restrictions are not evident when the patient is lying relaxed on the table. Often there is full pain-free neck rotation when the therapist passively moves the neck.

Central sensitization suggests that the experience of stiffness/pain during active movement or even manual stretching may be due solely to stretch sensitivity. It also implies that in some conditions ROM recovery can come about solely by desensitization (Fig. 9.4).

ROM DESENSITIZATION

The causes underlying the transition from acute to chronic sensitization are not fully understood. Factors associated with persistent sensitization include greater degree and longer duration of injury and genetic and psychosocial factors, to name but a few.[19,38] This means that preventing or removing the

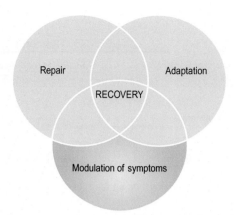

FIGURE 9.4 In some conditions, range of movement recovery can be primarily by desensitization.

cause of sensitization can be clinically elusive. The central nature of sensitization makes it even more elusive for physical therapies since there is nothing to "fix" peripherally in the tissues. All this suggests that to promote desensitization we need to focus on central process, somehow engaging the potential adaptive capacity of the nociceptive systems.

Before we set out to promote desensitization we have to establish in which conditions it will be beneficial.

When is ROM desensitization beneficial?

Whether ROM desensitization is beneficial depends on the role of pain within the patient's condition. An important consideration is whether pain/sensitization serves a protective function, which is partly related to the duration of the patient's condition, i.e. whether the condition is acute or persistent (Fig. 9.5).

Acute condition – In acute conditions pain and sensitization are likely to be part of a protective strategy. In these conditions the subjective experience of stiffness may be due to localized swelling and sensitization. Improvement in pain and ROM sensitization are often spontaneous and related to the rate of tissue healing.[39] Therefore, desensitization is not a therapeutic priority and the focus should be on assisting tissue repair. During that period the patient should be advised to remain active and ROM challenges should be within tolerable pain ranges. Furthermore, acute injuries are associated with tearing/damage of fibres and reduced tensile strength rather than structural shortening of tissues (Fig. 9.6). Therefore, end-range challenges may be unnecessary and unsafe in recently acquired injuries.

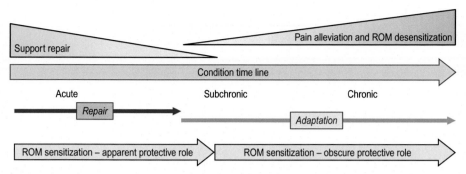

FIGURE 9.5 To desensitize or not: depends on the role of pain/sensitization in the condition. It may be more beneficial in persistent sensitization in which pain no longer provides a protective function. ROM, range of movement.

This raises the question of how long a condition is considered to be acute and when should the ROM challenges be introduced. Generally, tissue inflammation and regeneration are most marked within the first 2 weeks of injury. This duration may depend on the magnitude of damage and the type of tissue injured. A safety margin of 3–6 weeks is a useful time scale to consider a condition as acute.[40] Indeed, in many injuries or post-operative conditions the repair processes will resolve within this time frame.

However, pain relief, rather than optimized tissue healing, is often the patient's priority (most patients are not aware that inflammation is a positive aspect of repair). Some transient pain relief could be obtained by helping to minimize oedema and inflammatory by-products. Both of these therapeutic goals (healing and pain relief) can be achieved by the use of rhythmic movement

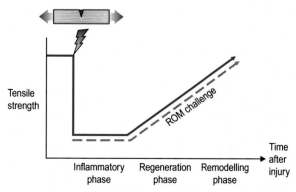

FIGURE 9.6 Tissue tensile strength following injury may be reduced. Range of movement (ROM) challenges should not exceed these levels.

(active or passive) and external intermittent compression within pain-free ranges (for full exploration of this topic see Lederman[41]).[42,43] Stretching is unlikely to have a positive influence on these processes.[41]

So, in acute conditions, ROM recovery can come about primarily by repair processes (Fig. 9.7).

Chronic conditions – ROM desensitization can be beneficial in persistent musculo-skeletal conditions. Here there is no obvious protective function for pain and sensitization (since there is an absence of tissue damage/inflammation). However, this clinical reasoning can be a bit more complicated; in asymptomatic, pain-free individuals it is common to find tissue damage without inflammation. For example, partial or full rotator cuff tears can be found in 34% of asymptomatic individuals.[44] Similarly, in the spine, the prevalence of tissue damage in asymptomatic individuals can be fairly high: 27% disc protrusion, 54% disc degeneration and 28% annular tears.[45] This means that tissue damage without pain is a fairly common occurrence. Another consideration is that pain does not always reflect the magnitude of tissue damage.[46] For example, non-perforated rotator cuff tears can be more painful than full-thickness tears.[47,48] In the spine, the degree of disc displacement, nerve root enhancement or nerve compression does not correlate with the magnitude of pain or disability.[49] It means that in more chronic conditions *the pain experience is (often) disproportionate or even unrelated to the underlying tissue damage.*

This brings us back to the original question: whether ROM challenges would be safe for chronic conditions in which "old" tissue damage is accompanied by pain/sensitization. In the spinal and shoulder conditions described above physical activities/exercise are considered to be both safe and beneficial for improvement/recovery.[50-60] From this it can be loosely concluded that, in

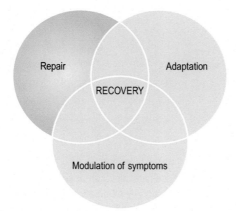

FIGURE 9.7 In some conditions ROM recovery can be primarily from tissue repair.

chronic conditions in which there is pain and potential underlying "old damage", ROM challenges are both safe and likely to be beneficial.

This leaves us with the question of how physical therapy can facilitate ROM desensitization.

Factors supporting ROM desensitization

Neural inhibitory mechanisms are inherent in all brain functions, including in the transmission of nociception and in desensitization processes.[61] Physical therapies often aim to exploit these inhibitory mechanisms in order to control/alleviate pain.

The modulation of nociception/pain can be largely by psychological/cognitive/emotional processes and partly by the physical sensory stimulation components of the treatment (Fig. 9.8). Although these mechanisms can be explored individually, in practice they are inseparable. It is difficult to specifically target one inhibitory system to the exclusion of another. Furthermore, the inhibition associated with desensitization is not exclusive to a particular aspect of the treatment, pathway or brain centre.[62-64] Pain alleviation and desensitization

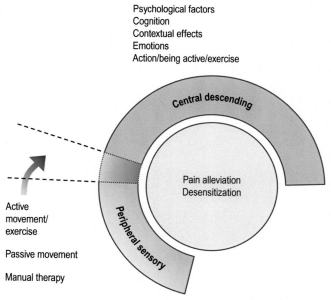

FIGURE 9.8 Pain alleviation and desensitization can arise by central descending inhibitory processes and peripherally induce inhibition by stimulation of mechanoreceptors. Peripheral mechanisms can modulate nociceptive transmission but also may be associated with descending inhibition through contextual effects (overlap area).

should be considered as whole-person responses to the entire therapeutic encounter – psychological and physical.[65]

Psychological dimension

Therapies that target psychological factors are known to have a potent influence on the experience of pain and sensitization.[62,66] The main psychological factors which may help mediate desensitization can be divided into three broad areas: emotional, cognitive and contextual factors.

Emotional factors

Sensitization and the experience of pain can be heightened by negative mood changes, such as depression, distress, anxiety and fear, whereas improvements in psychological well-being are often associated with alleviation of pain.[67–73] When patients with lower back pain experience negative moods they tend to report an increase in pain levels and decreased pain tolerance, with positive moods having the opposite effect.[74] This suggests that therapeutic interventions that help to improve psychological well-being may also have a positive impact on the pain experience.

There is a link between physical activities and a positive change in various psychological factors.[75] Even (the humble) walking can have a positive influence on psychological factors such as depression,[76] but also on chronic back pain.[77–79] One way to exploit the links between physical activity, psychological well-being and pain is to encourage the patient to return to physical activities, particularly those that they enjoy.[80]

Cognitive–behavioural factors

The patient's experience of pain and degrees of sensitization can be influenced by anxieties associated with their condition. Anxieties are often expressed as fears about movement, with the patient making inexact and disproportionate links between physical activities and the potential for greater pain and recurrence of injury (*catastrophizing*). When such anxieties were present, they were shown to have a negative influence on the experience of pain.[37,80–86] For example, patients who have a higher catastrophizing score before surgery tend to experience more pain following surgery.[82,87] Conversely, a decrease in pain catastrophizing can bring about a reduction in pain intensity and disability.[88,89]

These anxieties/fears can be alleviated by providing positive messages that reduce catastrophizing, empower the patient and promote self-efficacy in pain control.[89] It is useful to provide information about the nature of sensitization, highlighting the disparity between tissue damage and pain and the potential to modulate the pain experience through various cognitive and behavioural means (Ch. 11).[89,90] A patient with a chronic lower back condition who presents with ROM stiffness/discomfort can be informed that the area may be sensitive but not necessarily damaged, that discomfort experienced during or after movement in certain ranges does not mean that the spine has been re-damaged, and so on. These messages can be delivered explicitly and cognitively by verbal communication, but equally by "unspoken" messages that are conveyed implicitly by positive physical experiences (see reassurance, Ch. 11). This could explain why outcomes are similar for physical and cognitive–behavioural therapies in the treatment of chronic low back pain.[35,91-94] It has been proposed that the improvements in both groups are mediated by alleviating the anxieties associated with pain.

Pain experiences can also be alleviated by diverting attention away from the area of pain.[95-100] This can be done by drawing attention to another part of the body or to a particular mental or non-painful physical task.[101] The immediate application of this clinically is to provide movement strategies that emphasize an external focus of attention. This can be towards an external goal or outcome of a task rather than focusing on the painful area. For example, patients with chronic low back pain can be instructed to perform reaching movements, at end-range, while focusing on the target rather than on the discomfort in the back ("forget the back therapy").

Within the cognitive–behavioural dimension, relaxation techniques also have an important role in helping to control acute and chronic pain conditions.[102-109] Relaxation techniques can help distract attention from pain, support an internal locus of control and improve self-efficacy in managing pain.[107,108] Simple relaxation techniques, such as progressive muscle relaxation, have been found to be effective in managing chronic pain.[107,108,110]

Contextual effects

Contextual effects are the environmental factors which influence the patient's perception of the treatment. These factors can have a profound lasting effect on the patient's experience of pain.[111-115] Often, these factors are not directly associated with the physical aspect of the treatment but associated with the therapeutic relationship,[116] the patient's expectations, previous therapeutic experiences, treatment credibility and the patient's preference for a particular treatment.[35,92,94,111-113,117-119] When these contextual factors are positive they provide the individual with internal narratives that engage them psychologically, behaviourally and physiologically in their recovery.[114]

Contextual effects can have a significant influence on neurophysiological processes including sensitization/desensitization.[120] For example, the individual's expectation of pain, or, conversely, of pain relief, can determine the magnitude of spinal sensitization.[121] This was demonstrated in a study in which hypersensitivity to mechanical stimulation was induced by heating the skin of the forearm.[121] The area of sensitization was smaller in subjects who received a placebo analgesic in the form of a sham magnet (a metal plate shaped like a magnet applied to the sensitive area). Brain and spinal imaging during such placebo analgesia has demonstrated that the subject's report of reduced pain coincides with decreased activity in the brain pain areas with a concurrent inhibition of nociceptive input within the spinal cord.[115,120] There is some evidence that contextual effects on pain are more prominent in treatments that contain physical events, such as manual therapy, than in interventions where medication or psychological approaches are used.[122]

Physical components
Active movement

Active movement challenges can also play a role in ROM desensitization. Several studies have explored the effects of exercise on induced pain in healthy individuals.[123] Transient desensitization has been demonstrated during and after different forms of exercise. In dynamic, aerobic exercise desensitization is more likely to occur when the exercise is performed for more than 10 minutes and at above 70% of maximal aerobic capacity.[124-126] For isometric exercise it seems that less effort and duration is required for desensitization to take place.[63,127,128] It can be observed at an intensity as low as 25% of full contraction force and within a period of time as brief as 1 minute.[129,130]

Reduced hypersensitivity to activity has also been demonstrated in patients with chronic musculoskeletal conditions. In tennis elbow, active wrist movement combined with superimposed elbow joint mobilization demonstrated an immediate reduction in sensitization.[26-28] Similarly, in patients with chronic neck pain, 3 minutes of specific neck exercises, performed in non-painful ranges, was shown to reduce local hypersensitivity and improve cervical pain-free ranges.[131] Overall, these studies demonstrate that active forms of ROM challenges could be useful for inducing desensitization. This could be achieved both by rhythmic, cyclical movement and by static isometric-like activities. These challenges should be applied within the pain-free ranges of movement.

These principles can be applied clinically within the framework of a functional approach. For example, a patient with chronic low back pain can be instructed to perform a repetitive reaching movement, towards a target marked by the therapist's hand. The procedure starts by exploring the patient's pain-free range by moving the target hand to different positions. Once a comfortable sphere of movement is established the patient repeats the reaching movement towards these positions. After several reaching cycles the therapist surreptitiously moves the target hand further away. If there is no pain at the new position the patient is instructed to repeat the movement to this range, and so on (see accompanying Video).

Passive movement and stretching

A wide range of manual therapy approaches use passive techniques to control pain and reduce sensitization. These include stretching, massage, manipulation and joint mobilization/articulation.

Passive manual approaches base their analgesic influences on the capacity of proprioceptors to modulate nociceptive signals (pain-gate phenomenon).[132–134] In one of the early studies of the pain-gate mechanism it was demonstrated that a noxious stimulus of the cat's paw can be modulated, in the spinal cord, by a simultaneous application of vibration to the paw (proprioceptive stimulus).[133] A similar phenomenon was later demonstrated in humans.[133] A special vibrator with a ring applicator was placed on the skin of the thigh and a noxious stimulus was applied through the centre of the ring. When the vibrator was switched on the subject experienced less pain and had difficulty in localizing it. However, the pain returned once the vibrator was switched off. A similar phenomenon was demonstrated with induced muscle pain (injection of an irritant into the muscle) and passive movement of a nearby joint.[135] During passive motion there was an immediate decrease in muscle pain (17–31%) and point pressure pain (17%). This desensitization by passive movement was also demonstrated in animals with chronic muscle and joint inflammation; mobilization of a nearby joint reduced the sensitization in the affected areas.[136]

This gating phenomenon was also demonstrated in manual therapy studies. Passive techniques applied remotely or close to the area of sensitization were shown to bring about immediate desensitization.[135,137,138] This has also been shown by various studies of spinal manipulation (which can be considered as a very rapid stretch at the end-range). A single manipulation has been shown to produce some form of desensitization segmentally at the spine and even distally in the limbs.[137,138]

Overall, it seems that desensitization is more likely to occur during dynamic rather than static stretching events.[132–138] This is probably due to the presence of a sustained proprioceptive barrage during dynamic events (Fig. 9.9). An example of dynamic stretching is passive cyclical joint oscillation/mobilization at end-ranges, such as a pendular swing of the limb/segment within the pain-free ranges. A gating effect is likely to be minimal during static stretching owing to a drop in the sensory barrage (static receptors are fast adapting and tend to be less numerous than dynamic receptors).

Transient nature of desensitization

There are two physiological hurdles that need to be overcome for desensitization to be successful. The first is the transient nature of a physically induced

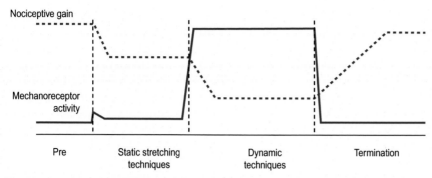

FIGURE 9.9 Gating of nociceptive transmission by mechanoreceptor stimulation. Greater inhibition is expected during dynamic manual events. However at termination of stimulation nociception is expected to return to pre-session levels, unless maintained by descending inhibitory influences.

desensitization and the second is the neural plasticity associated with sensitization.

Pain relief and desensitization are likely to be significant only as long as the physical stimulation is present, with perhaps some transient after-effect.[63,139–141] For example, desensitization after exercise tends to taper off within 30 minutes after termination of the activity.[126,128,139] This may be even more critical for passive approaches in which inhibition depends on ongoing proprioceptive stimulation. It would be expected that desensitization would rapidly decrease during static events, such as at the termination of the dynamic phase of stretching or passive movement (Fig. 9.7). Desensitization that outlasts its physical stimulation is more likely to depend on sustained central inhibition from higher centres, i.e. contextual effects/placebos (see above).

The second hurdle is the competition between the short duration of therapeutic intervention and the persistent adaptive nature of sensitization. Chronic sensitization shares the same neurological processes that underlie learning.[142,143] It is associated with robust anatomical and physiological plasticity within the peripheral and central nervous systems.[18,142–144] The consequence is a physiological competition between the persistence of sensitization and the transient nature of the therapeutic intervention. The winner of this competition is likely to be the persistent state of sensitization: it is there all the time.

To overcome the problem of duration and competition we need to explore, with the patient, inhibitory processes that are both persistent and self-sustaining. The most realistic approach is to engage the patient in psychological and cognitive processes, in particular reducing anxieties and promoting self-efficacy and self-care,[118] part of which can be exercise and relaxation. There are two other less favourable options – to identify and "remove" the pathological processes that maintain the sensitization or to increase the frequency of intervention. However, it can be difficult to identify the processes that maintain the sensitization and even more so to remove it. Increasing the frequency of treatment can be impractical and may even have negative consequences; as was shown in the management of whiplash injuries, too much treatment can promote chronicity and dependency.[145,146]

STRETCHING AND PAIN CONTROL

One of the most common uses of stretching is to alleviate pain after exercise and injury and to control chronic musculoskeletal pain.

In sports and exercise, stretching is often used before and after training to relieve delayed onset muscle soreness (DOMS). Although frequently used, it is largely ineffective in reducing pain. Stretching before exercise has been estimated to reduce DOMS by 1 point on a 100-point scale and stretching after exercise is estimated to reduce it by 0.5 on the 100-point scale.[147,148]

Since stretching is ineffective for DOMS, which is a mild/benign form of muscular damage, it is unlikely to provide pain relief in more severe musculoskeletal injuries. In acute and sub-acute low back pain, stretching does not seem to add any benefit above the advice to keep active.[149] Stretching may even be harmful in acute conditions where there is tissue damage and where pain serves a protection strategy (see above). For example, passive stretching after rotator cuff repair surgery resulted in a greater number of re-tears (23%) than pain-free passive motion (8%).[150]

Stretching exercise to alleviate chronic pain has shown mixed results.[151] A recent review suggests that yoga may provide some alleviation in various musculoskeletal and other pain conditions:[152,153] labour pain,[154] hand osteoarthritis,[155] migraine,[156] carpal tunnel syndrome[157] and irritable bowel syndrome.[158] In particular for chronic low back pain, several studies have demonstrated greater pain relief with yoga than with other forms of exercise or standard care.[159–162] However, in yoga other elements of practice may also influence pain levels, such as raised self-efficacy, relaxation and breathing exercise. A recent large study with 228 subjects compared 12 weeks of yoga, conventional stretching exercises and self-care information for chronic low back pain.[163] Both yoga and stretching resulted in similar pain reductions that lasted several months; however, this effect seems to be modest and did not reach clinical significance.[163] In another recent study, six sessions of yoga had no effect on low back pain.[164]

For chronic, non-specific neck pain regular stretching exercise shows mixed results.[151] Some studies show pain reduction in the short term (4–12 weeks),[165,166] some show improvement in the long term when intensively maintained with other forms of exercise,[167] while others have not demonstrated any additional benefit.[168-171]

One study has demonstrated that stretching may increase sensitization of tender points in patients with various musculoskeletal pain conditions.[172]

In a systematic review carried out in 2010, stretching was shown to have no effect on pain levels in subjects who experience pain and loss of ROM due to various musculoskeletal, neurological and surgical complications.[173]

CLINICAL REASONING IN ROM REHABILITATION IN THE PRESENCE OF PAIN

With all the information discussed above we can now return to the case scenarios described at the beginning of this chapter and explore the clinical reasoning for management (Fig. 9.10):

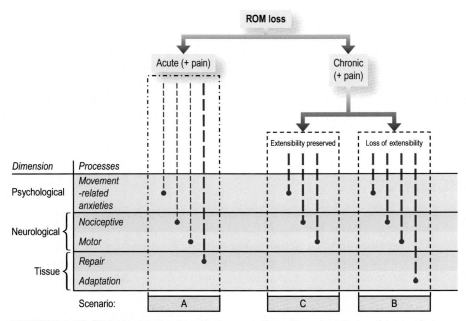

FIGURE 9.10 Clinical reasoning in patients presenting with various forms of range of movement (ROM) loss in the presence of pain. Heavier dashed lines imply prioritizing.

Patient A presents with a knee sprain which happened 1 week ago. It is painful, swollen and stiff and on examination has only a limited ROM.

In this clinical scenario the priority is to support the tissue repair processes. It is estimated that ROM sensitization and pain will subside as the condition improves. This can be achieved by a variety of passive and active movement approaches. Stretching (tissue overloading) is not indicated and may be unsafe in this case.

Patient B had a knee joint fracture. It is now 6 weeks later and the plaster has just been removed. The knee is painful, swollen, has restricted ROM and is very stiff.

In this case, the focus is on all three dimensions. The priority, however, is in the tissue dimension promoting local adaptive recovery of ROM but with an emphasis on active challenges to recover motor control (neurological dimension). Pain alleviation and desensitization can be both engaged in the psychological (e.g. reducing the condition-related anxieties) and neurological (e.g. modulation of symptoms using dynamic movement approaches) dimensions.

Here, tissue repair is likely to have been resolved. Overloading of tissue, although uncomfortable, is likely to be safe and even beneficial.

Patient C had a knee surgery 1 year ago. On examination the passive knee ranges have mostly recovered but pain and stiffness are still limiting the patient's functional ranges.

In this clinical scenario the priority is to reduce ROM sensitization, processes that are predominantly in the psychological–neurological dimensions. Here, tissue loading/stretching is unlikely to be beneficial for recovery (no point in stretching something which is not shortened). Varying levels of pain alleviation and desensitization can be achieved by the methods discussed throughout this chapter (see also psychological consideration, Ch. 11).

SUMMARY

- Sensitization is a neurological process in which the central nervous system can change, distort or amplify the experience of pain
- ROM sensitization is a neurological process in which pain, discomfort or stiffness are experienced in normal ROM
- In acute conditions, sensitization and pain have a positive protective role in limiting the ROM
- In acute conditions, stretching or challenging end-ranges is unlikely to be useful and may even increase the likelihood of re-injury. The therapeutic focus should be on supporting recovery

- In some conditions, ROM recovery may be associated primarily with teh repair process
- In chronic conditions, ROM sensitization can be the primary cause of ROM losses; it can be present in the absence of inflammation, tissue damage or tissue shortening
- Desensitization is likely to be useful and beneficial in chronic conditions, in which pain and sensitivity have no obvious protective function
- In persistent conditions, ROM recovery may come about primarily by symptomatic relief and desensitization
- ROM sensitivity can be reduced by approaches that incorporate psychological and physical means
- Alleviating the condition-related anxieties is one of the key components in managing pain in the psychological–behavioural dimension
- Psychological and behavioural means are more likely to provide/sustain long-term desensitization and pain alleviation
- Stretching techniques are ineffective in managing acute pain. It is unclear whether stretching is useful for chronic pain; if it has an effect it is likely to be modest
- Pain processes are part of complex systems that produce complex responses; the outcome can be variable, disproportionate and unpredictable in relation to the therapeutic intervention

REFERENCES

1. Woolf CJ. Central sensitization: implications for the diagnosis and treatment of pain. Pain 2011;152(3 Suppl):S2–15.
2. Grubb BD. Activation of sensory neurons in the arthritic joint. Novartis Found Symp 2004;260:28–36.
3. Woolf CJ, Ma Q. Nociceptors: noxious stimulus detectors. Neuron 2007;55(3):353–64.
4. Wang H, Ehnert C, Brenner GJ, et al. Bradykinin and peripheral sensitization. Biol Chem 2006;387(1):11–14.
5. Schaible H-G, Grubb BD. Afferents and spinal mechanisms of joint pain. Pain 1993;55: 5–54.
6. Coggeshall RE, Hong KAHP, Langford LA, et al. Discharge characteristics of fine medial articular afferents at rest and during passive movement of the inflamed knee joints. Brain Res 1983;272:185–8.
7. Radhakrishnan R, Moore SA, Sluka KA. Unilateral carrageenan injection into muscle or joint induces chronic bilateral hyperalgesia in rats. Pain 2003;104:567–77.
8. Neugebauer V, Schaible HG. Evidence for a central component in the sensitization of spinal neurons with joint input during development of acute arthritis in cat's knee. J Neurophysiol 1990;64:299–311.
9. Lenz FA, Lee JI, Garonzik IM, et al. Plasticity of pain-related neuronal activity in the human thalamus. Prog Brain Res 2000;129:259–73.
10. Dubner R, Basbaum AI. Spinal dorsal horn plasticity following tissue or nerve injury. In: Wall PD, Melzack R, editors. Textbook of pain. 3rd ed. London: Churchill Livingstone; 1994:225–42.
11. Cervero F, Laird JM, Garcia-Nicas E. Secondary hyperalgesia and presynaptic inhibition: an update. Eur J Pain 2003;7(4):345–51.

12. Woolf CJ. The dorsal horn: state-dependent sensory processing and the generation of pain. In: Wall PD, Melzack R, editors. Textbook of pain. 3rd ed. London: Churchill Livingstone; 1994:101–12.
13. Wilder-Smith OH, Tassonyi E, Arendt-Nielsen L. Preoperative back pain is associated with diverse manifestations of central neuroplasticity. Pain 2002;97(3):189–94.
14. Cook AJ, Woolf CJ, Wall PD, et al. Dynamic receptive field plasticity in rat spinal dorsal horn following C-primary afferent input. Nature 1987;325:151–3.
15. Hylden JLK, Nahin RL, Traub RJ, et al. Expansion of receptive fields of spinal lamina I projection neurons in rat with unilateral adjuvant-induced inflammation: the contribution of dorsal horn mechanisms. Pain 1989;37:229–43.
16. Dunbar R, Ruda MA. Activity-dependent neuronal plasticity following tissue injury and inflammation. Trends Neurosci 1992;15(3):96–103.
17. Ordeberg G. Characterization of joint pain in human OA. Novartis Found Symp 2004;260: 105–15.
18. Woolf CJ. Central sensitization: uncovering the relation between pain and plasticity. Anesthesiology 2007;106(4):864–7.
19. Schnabel A, Pogatzki-Zahn E. Predictors of chronic pain following surgery. What do we know? Schmerz 2010;24(5):517–31.
20. Curatolo M, Petersen-Felix S, Arendt-Nielsen L, et al. Central hypersensitivity in chronic pain after whiplash injury. Clin J Pain 2001;17(4):306–15.
21. Bajaj P, Graven-Nielsen T, Arendt-Nielsen L. Osteoarthritis and its association with muscle hyperalgesia: an experimental controlled study. Pain 2001;93(2):107–14.
22. Gerdle B, Hilgenfeldt U, Larsson B, et al. Bradykinin and kallidin levels in the trapezius muscle in patients with work-related trapezius myalgia, in patients with whiplash associated pain, and in healthy controls: a microdialysis study of women. Pain 2008;139(3):578–87.
23. Koelbaek Johansen M. Generalised muscular hyperalgesia in chronic whiplash syndrome. Pain 1999;83(2):229–34.
24. Rosendale L, Larsson B, Kristiansen J, et al. Increase in muscle nociceptive substances and anaerobic metabolism in patients with trapezius myalgia: microdialysis in rest and during exercise. Pain 2004;112:324–34.
25. Sjøgaard G, Rosendal L, Kristiansen J, et al. Muscle oxygenation and glycolysis in females with trapezius myalgia during stress and repetitive work using microdialysis and NIRS. Eur J Appl Physiol 2010;108(4):657–69.
26. Abbott JH, Patla CE, Jensen RH. The initial effects of an elbow mobilization with movement technique on grip strength in subjects with lateral epicondylalgia. Man Ther 2001;6(3): 163–9.
27. Paungmali A, Vicenzino B, Smith M. Hypoalgesia induced by elbow manipulation in lateral epicondylalgia does not exhibit tolerance. J Pain 2003;4(8):448–54.
28. Paungmali A, O'Leary S, Souvlis T, et al. Hypoalgesic and sympathoexcitatory effects of mobilization with movement for lateral epicondylalgia. Phys Ther 2003;83(4):374–83.
29. van Wilgen CP, Keizer D. Neuropathic pain mechanisms in patients with chronic sports injuries: a diagnostic model useful in sports medicine? Pain Med 2011;12(1):110–17.
30. van Wilgen CP, Konopka KH, Keizer D, et al. Do patients with chronic patellar tendinopathy have an altered somatosensory profile? A Quantitative Sensory Testing (QST) study. Scand J Med Sci Sports 2013;23(2):149–55.
31. Fernández-Carnero J, Fernández-de-Las-Peñas C, de la Llave-Rincón AI, et al. Widespread mechanical pain hypersensitivity as sign of central sensitization in unilateral epicondylalgia: a blinded, controlled study. Clin J Pain 2009;25(7):555–61.
32. Schaible HG, Richter F, Ebersberger A, et al. Joint pain. Exp Brain Res 2009;196(1):153–62.
33. Halbertsma JP, Göeken LN, Hof AL, et al. Extensibility and stiffness of the hamstrings in patients with nonspecific low back pain. Arch Phys Med Rehabil 2001;82(2):232–8.
34. Esola MA, McClure PW, Fitzgerald GK, et al. Analysis of lumbar spine and hip motion during forward bending in subjects with and without a history of low back pain. Spine 1996;21(1): 71–8.

35. Johnson RE, Jones GT, Wiles NJ, et al. Active exercise, education, and cognitive behavioral therapy for persistent disabling low back pain: a randomized controlled trial. Spine 2007;32(15):1578–85.

36. Hultman G, Saraste H, Ohlsen H. Anthropometry, spinal canal width, and flexibility of the spine and hamstring muscles in 45–55-year-old men with and without low back pain. J Spinal Disord 1992;5(3):245–53.

37. Sullivan MS, Shoaf LD, Riddle DL. The relationship of lumbar flexion to disability in patients with low back pain. Phys Ther 2000;80(3):240–50.

38. Kehlet H, Jensen TS, Woolf CJ. Persistent postsurgical pain: risk factors and prevention. Lancet 2006;367(9522):1618–25.

39. Hildebrandt J. Does unspecific low back pain really exist? Z Orthop Ihre Grenzgeb 2004;142(2):139–45.

40. van Tulder M, Malmivaara A, Esmail R, et al. Exercise therapy for low back pain: a systematic review within the framework of the Cochrane Collaboration Back Review Group. Spine 2000;25(21):2784–96.

41. Lederman E. The science and practice of manual therapy. Edinburgh: Elsevier; 2005.

42. Butterfield TA, Zhao Y, Agarwal S, et al. Cyclic compressive loading facilitates recovery after eccentric exercise. Med Sci Sports Exerc 2008;40(7):1289–96.

43. Jakeman JR, Byrne C, Eston RG. Lower limb compression garment improves recovery from exercise-induced muscle damage in young, active females. Eur J Appl Physiol 2010;109(6): 1137–44.

44. Sher JS, Uribe JW, Posada A, et al. Abnormal findings on magnetic resonance images of asymptomatic shoulders. J Bone Joint Surg Am 1995;77(1):10–15.

45. Endean A, Palmer KT, Coggon D. Potential of magnetic resonance imaging findings to refine case definition for mechanical low back pain in epidemiological studies. Spine 2011;36(2): 160–9.

46. Lederman E. The fall of the postural-structural-biomechanical model in manual and physical therapies: exemplified by lower back pain. J Bodyw Mov Ther 2011;15(2):131–8.

47. Gotoh M, Hamada K, Yamakawa H, et al. Increased substance P in subacromial bursa and shoulder pain in rotator cuff diseases. J Orthop Res 1998;16(5):618–21.

48. McCabe RA, Nicholas SJ, Montgomery KD, et al. The effect of rotator cuff tear size on shoulder strength and range of motion. J Orthop Sports Phys Ther 2005;35(3):130–5.

49. Karppinen J, Malmivaara A, Tervonen O, et al. Severity of symptoms and signs in relation to magnetic resonance imaging findings among sciatic patients. Spine 2001;26(7):E149–54.

50. Itoi E, Tabata S. Conservative treatment of rotator cuff tears. Clin Orthop Relat Res 1992;275: 165–73.

51. Brox JI, Staff PH, Ljunggren AE, et al. Arthroscopic surgery compared with supervised exercises in patients with rotator cuff disease (stage II impingement syndrome). Br Med J 1993;307(6909):899–903.

52. Morrison DS, Frogameni AD, Woodworth P. Non-operative treatment of subacromial impingement syndrome. J Bone Joint Surg 1997;79(5):732–7.

53. Battié MC. Volvo Award in Clinical Sciences. Determinants of lumbar disc degeneration: a study relating lifetime exposures and magnetic resonance imaging findings in identical twins. Spine 1995;20(24):2601–12.

54. Videman T. Determinants of the progression in lumbar degeneration: a 5-year follow-up study of adult male monozygotic twins. Spine 2006;31(6):671–8.

55. Carragee E, Alamin T, Cheng I, et al. Does minor trauma cause serious low back illness? Spine 2006;31(25):2942–9.

56. Bakker EW, Verhagen AP, van Trijffel E, et al. Spinal mechanical load as a risk factor for low back pain: a systematic review of prospective cohort studies. Spine 2009;34(8):E281–93.

57. Roffey DM, Wai EK, Bishop P, et al. Causal assessment of awkward occupational postures and low back pain: results of a systematic review. Spine J 2010;10:89–99.

58. Wai EK, Roffey DM, Bishop P, et al. Causal assessment of occupational bending or twisting and low back pain: results of a systematic review. Spine J 2010;10:76–88.

59. Waddell G, Burton AK. Occupational health guidelines for the management of low back pain at work: evidence review. Occup Med 2001;51(2):124–35.
60. Hilde G, Hagen KB, Jamtvedt G, Winnem M. Advice to stay active as a single treatment for low back pain and sciatica. Cochrane Database Syst Rev 2007;3:CD003632.
61. Melzack R. From the gate to the neuromatrix. Pain 1999;6(Suppl):S121–6.
62. Goffaux P, Redmond WJ, Rainville P, et al. Descending analgesia: when the spine echoes what the brain expects. Pain 2007;130(1–2):137–43.
63. Pertovaara A, Kemppainen P, Leppänen H. Lowered cutaneous sensitivity to nonpainful electrical stimulation during isometric exercise in humans. Exp Brain Res 1992;89(2):447–52.
64. Schweinhardt P, Bushnell MC. Pain imaging in health and disease: how far have we come? J Clin Invest 2010;120(11):3788–97.
65. Colloca L, Benedetti F. How prior experience shapes placebo analgesia. Pain 2006;124(1–2):126–33.
66. Palermo TM, Eccleston C, Lewandowski AS, et al. Randomized controlled trials of psychological therapies for management of chronic pain in children and adolescents: an updated meta-analytic review. Pain 2010;148(3):387–97.
67. Berna C, Leknes S, Holmes EA, et al. Induction of depressed mood disrupts emotion regulation neurocircuitry and enhances pain unpleasantness. Biol Psychiatry 2010;67(11):1083–90.
68. Villemure C, Bushnell MC. Mood influences supraspinal pain processing separately from attention. J Neurosci 2009;29(3):705–15.
69. Owen DG, Clarke CF, Ganapathy S, et al. Using perfusion MRI to measure the dynamic changes in neural activation associated with tonic muscular pain. Pain 2010;148(3):375–86.
70. Hiebert R, Campello MA, Weiser S, et al. Predictors of short-term work-related disability among active duty US Navy personnel: a cohort study in patients with acute and subacute low back pain. Spine J 2012;12(9):806–16.
71. Pincus T, Burton AK, Vogel S, et al. A systematic review of psychological factors as predictors of chronicity/disability in prospective cohorts of low back pain. Spine 2002;27(5):E109–20.
72. Pincus T, Vogel S, Burton AK, et al. Fear avoidance and prognosis in back pain: a systematic review and synthesis of current evidence. Arthritis Rheum 2006;54(12):3999–4010.
73. George SZ, Wittmer VT, Fillingim RB, et al. Sex and pain-related psychological variables are associated with thermal pain sensitivity for patients with chronic low back pain. J Pain 2007;8(1):2–10.
74. Tang NK, Salkovskis PM, Hodges A, et al. Effects of mood on pain responses and pain tolerance: an experimental study in chronic back pain patients. Pain 2008;138(2):392–401.
75. Steptoe A, Edwards S, Moses J. The effects of exercise training on mood and perceived coping ability in anxious adults from the general population. J Psychosom Res 1989;33(5):537–47.
76. Cutshaw CA, Staten LK, Reinschmidt KM, et al. Depressive symptoms and health-related quality of life among participants in the Pasos Adelante Chronic Disease Prevention and Control Program, Arizona, 2005–2008. Prev Chronic Dis 2008;9:E24.
77. Olaya-Contreras P, Styf J, Lundberg M, et al. Cross-validation of the Depression, Anxiety, and Positive Outlook Scale (DAPOS) for clinical use. Clin J Pain 2011;27(4):330–7.
78. Smeets RJ. Do lumbar stabilising exercises reduce pain and disability in patients with recurrent low back pain? Aust J Physiother 2009;55(2):138.
79. Little P, Lewith G, Webley F, et al. Randomised controlled trial of Alexander technique lessons, exercise, and massage (ATEAM) for chronic and recurrent back pain. Br Med J 2008;337:a884.
80. Sullivan MJ, Stanish W, Waite H, et al. Catastrophizing, pain, and disability in patients with soft-tissue injuries. Pain 1998;77(3):253–60.

81. Sullivan MJ, Stanish W, Sullivan ME, et al. Differential predictors of pain and disability in patients with whiplash injuries. Pain Res Manag 2002;7(2):68–74.
82. Pavlin DJ, Sullivan MJ, Freund PR, et al. Catastrophizing: a risk factor for postsurgical pain. Clin J Pain 2005;21:83–90.
83. Keefe FJ, Lefebvre JC, Egert JR, et al. The relationship of gender to pain, pain behavior, and disability in osteoarthritis patients: the role of catastrophising. Pain 2000;87:325–34.
84. Walton DM, Pretty J, MacDermid JC, et al. Risk factors for persistent problems following whiplash injury: results of a systematic review and meta-analysis. J Orthop Sports Phys Ther 2009;39(5):334–50.
85. Goodin BR, McGuire L, Allshouse M, et al. Associations between catastrophizing and endogenous pain-inhibitory processes: sex differences. J Pain 2009;10(2):180–90.
86. Severeijns R, Vlaeyen JW, van den Hout MA, et al. Pain catastrophizing predicts pain intensity, disability, and psychological distress independent of the level of physical impairment. Clin J Pain 2001;17(2):165–72.
87. Khan RS, Ahmed K, Blakeway E, et al. Catastrophizing: a predictive factor for postoperative pain. Am J Surg 2011;201(1):122–31.
88. Smeets RJ, Vlaeyen JW, Kester AD, et al. Reduction of pain catastrophizing mediates the outcome of both physical and cognitive-behavioral treatment in chronic low back pain. J Pain 2006;7(4):261–71.
89. Spinhoven P, Ter KM, Kole-Snijders AM, et al. Catastrophizing and internal pain control as mediators of outcome in the multidisciplinary treatment of chronic low back pain. Eur J Pain 2004;8(3):211–19.
90. Louw A, Diener I, Butler DS, et al. The effect of neuroscience education on pain, disability, anxiety, and stress in chronic musculoskeletal pain. Arch Phys Med Rehabil 2011;92: 2041–56.
91. Smeets RJ, Vlaeyen JW, Kester AD, et al. Reduction of pain catastrophizing mediates the outcome of both physical and cognitive-behavioral treatment in chronic low back pain. J Pain 2006;7(4):261–71.
92. Smeets RJ, Beelen S, Goossens ME, et al. Treatment expectancy and credibility are associated with the outcome of both physical and cognitive-behavioral treatment in chronic low back pain. Clin J Pain 2008;24(4):305–15.
93. Critchley DJ, Ratcliffe J, Noonan S, et al. Effectiveness and cost-effectiveness of three types of physiotherapy used to reduce chronic low back pain disability: a pragmatic randomized trial with economic evaluation. Spine 2007;32(14):1474–81.
94. Albaladejo C, Kovacs FM, Royuela A, et al. The efficacy of a short education program and a short physiotherapy program for treating low back pain in primary care: a cluster randomized trial. Spine 2010;35(5):483–96.
95. Bantick SJ, Wise RG, Ploghaus A, et al. Imaging how attention modulates pain in humans using functional MRI. Brain 2002;125(pt 2):310–19.
96. Brooks JC, Nurmikko TJ, Bimson WE, et al. fMRI of thermal pain: effects of stimulus laterality and attention. Neuroimage 2002;15(2):293–301.
97. Longe SE, Wise R, Bantick S, et al. Counter-stimulatory effects on pain perception and processing are significantly altered by attention: an fMRI study. Neuroreport 2001; 12(9):2021–5.
98. Valet M, Sprenger T, Boecker H, et al. Distraction modulates connectivity of the cingulo-frontal cortex and the midbrain during pain: an fMRI analysis. Pain 2004;109(3):399–408.
99. Wiech K, Seymour B, Kalisch R, et al. Modulation of pain processing in hyperalgesia by cognitive demand. Neuroimage 2005;27(1):59–69.
100. Sprenger C, Eippert F, Finsterbusch J, et al. Attention modulates spinal cord responses to pain. Curr Biol 2012;22(11):1019–22.
101. Schrooten MG, Van Damme S, Crombez G, et al. Nonpain goal pursuit inhibits attentional bias to pain. Pain 2012;153(6):1180–6.

102. Smith CA, Levett KM, Collins CT, et al. Relaxation techniques for pain management in labour. Cochrane Database Syst Rev 2011;12:CD009514.
103. Andersson G, Johansson C, Nordlander A, et al. Chronic pain in older adults: a controlled pilot trial of a brief cognitive-behavioural group treatment. Behav Cogn Psychother 2012; 239–44.
104. Kroner-Herwig B, Mohn U, Pothmann R. Comparison of biofeedback and relaxation in the treatment of pediatric headache and the influence of parent involvement on outcome. Appl Psychophysiol Biofeedback 1998;23:143–57.
105. Larsson B, Melin L. Chronic headaches in adolescents: treatment in a school setting with relaxation training as compared with information-contact and self-registration. Pain 1986;25:325–36.
106. Larsson B, Daleflod B, Hakansson L, et al. Therapist-assisted versus self-help relaxation treatment of chronic headaches in adolescents: a school-based intervention. J Child Psychol Psychiatry 1987;28:127–36.
107. Diezemann A. Relaxation techniques for chronic pain. Schmerz 2011;25(4):445–53.
108. Vlaeyen JW, Haazen IW, Schuerman JA, et al. Behavioural rehabilitation of chronic low back pain: comparison of an operant treatment, an operant-cognitive treatment and an operant-respondent treatment. Br J Clin Psychol 1995;34:95–118.
109. Morone NE, Greco CM. Mind–body interventions for chronic pain in older adults: a structured review. Pain Med 2007;8(4):359–75.
110. Kwekkeboom KL, Gretarsdottir E. Systematic review of relaxation interventions for pain. J Nurs Scholarsh 2006;38(3):269–77.
111. Colloca L, Tinazzi M, Recchia S, et al. Learning potentiates neurophysiological and behavioral placebo analgesic responses. Pain 2008;139(2):306–14.
112. Colloca L, Benedetti F. Placebo analgesia induced by social observational learning. Pain 2009;144(1–2):28–34.
113. Bialosky JE, Bishop MD, George SZ, et al. Placebo response to manual therapy: something out of nothing? J Man Manip Ther 2011;19(1):11–19.
114. Linde K, Fässler M, Meissner K. Placebo interventions, placebo effects and clinical practice. Phil. Trans. R. Soc. B 2011;366(1572):1905–12.
115. Eippert F, Finsterbusch J, Bingel U, et al. Direct evidence for spinal cord involvement in placebo analgesia. Science 2009;326(5951):404.
116. Miciak M, Gross DP, Joyce A. A review of the psychotherapeutic "common factors" model and its application in physical therapy: the need to consider general effects in physical therapy practice. Scand J Caring Sci 2012;26(2):394–403.
117. Bensing JM, Verheul W. The silent healer: the role of communication in placebo effects. Patient Educ Couns 2010;80(3):293–9.
118. Crow R, Gage H, Hampson S, et al. The role of expectancies in the placebo effect and their use in the delivery of health care: a systematic review. Health Technol Assess 1999;3(3):1–96.
119. Holm LW, Carroll LJ, Cassidy JD, et al. Expectations for recovery important in the prognosis of whiplash injuries. PLoS Med 2008;5(5):e105.
120. Bingel U. Mechanisms of endogenous pain modulation illustrated by placebo analgesia: functional imaging findings. Schmerz 2010;24(2):122–9.
121. Matre D, Casey KL, Knardahl S. Placebo-induced changes in spinal cord pain processing. J Neurosci 2006;26(2):559–63.
122. Hróbjartsson A, Gøtzsche PC. 2010. Placebo interventions for all clinical conditions. Cochrane Database Syst Rev 2006;1:CD003974.
123. Koltyn KF. Analgesia following exercise: a review. Sports Med 2000;29(2):85–98.
124. Anshel MH, Russell KG. Effect of aerobic and strength training on pain tolerance, pain appraisal and mood of unfit males as a function of pain location. J Sports Sci 1994;12(6):535–47.
125. Koltyn KF. Exercise-induced hypoalgesia and intensity of exercise. Sports Med 2002;32(8):477–87.

126. Hoffman MD, Shepanski MA, Ruble SB, et al. Intensity and duration threshold for aerobic exercise-induced analgesia to pressure pain. Arch Phys Med Rehabil 2004;85(7): 1183–7.

127. Koltyn KF, Umeda M. Contralateral attenuation of pain after short-duration submaximal isometric exercise. J Pain 2007;8(11):887–92.

128. Kosek E, Lundberg L. Segmental and plurisegmental modulation of pressure pain thresholds during static muscle contractions in healthy individuals. Eur J Pain 2003;7(3): 251–8.

129. Umeda M, Newcomb LW, Ellingson LD, et al. Examination of the dose–response relationship between pain perception and blood pressure elevations induced by isometric exercise in men and women. Biol Psychol 2010;85(1):90–6.

130. Focht BC, Koltyn KF. Alterations in pain perception after resistance exercise performed in the morning and evening. J Strength Cond Res 2009;23(3):891–7.

131. O'Leary S, Falla D, Hodges PW, et al. Specific therapeutic exercise of the neck induces immediate local hypoalgesia. J Pain 2007;8(11):832–9.

132. Melzack R, Wall PD. Pain mechanisms: a new theory. Science 1965;150(3699):971–9.

133. Wall PD, Cronly-Dillon JR. Pain, itch, and vibration. Arch Neurol 1960;2:365–75.

134. Ghez C, Lenzi GL. Modulation of lemniscal transmission during voluntary movement. Boll Soc Ital Biol Sper 1971;47(3):76–7.

135. Nielsen MM, Mortensen A, Sørensen JK, et al. Reduction of experimental muscle pain by passive physiological movements. Man Ther 2009;14(1):101–9.

136. Sluka KA, Skyba DA, Radhakrishnan R, et al. Joint mobilization reduces hyperalgesia associated with chronic muscle and joint inflammation in rats. J Pain 2006;7(8): 602–7.

137. Fernández-Carnero J, Fernández-de-las-Peñas C, Cleland JA. Immediate hypoalgesic and motor effects after a single cervical spine manipulation in subjects with lateral epicondylalgia. J Manip Physiol Ther 2008;31(9):675–81.

138. Fernández-Carnero J, Cleland JA, Arbizu RL. Examination of motor and hypoalgesic effects of cervical vs thoracic spine manipulation in patients with lateral epicondylalgia: a clinical trial. J Manip Physiol Ther 2011;34(7):432–40.

139. Paalasmaa P, Kemppainen P, Pertovaara A. Modulation of skin sensitivity by dynamic and isometric exercise in man. Eur J Appl Physiol Occup Physiol 1991;62(4):279–85.

140. Zoppi M, Voegelin MR, Signorini M, et al. Pain threshold changes by skin vibratory stimulation in healthy subjects. Acta Physiol Scand 1991;143(4):439–43.

141. Pantaleo T, Duranti R, Bellini F. Effects of vibratory stimulation on muscular pain threshold and blink response in human subjects. Pain 1986;24(2):239–50.

142. Laferrière A, Pitcher MH, Haldane A, et al. PKMζ is essential for spinal plasticity underlying the maintenance of persistent pain. Mol Pain 2011;7:99.

143. Ji RR, Kohno T, Moore KA, et al. Central sensitization and LTP: do pain and memory share similar mechanisms? Trends Neurosci 2003;26:696–705.

144. Flor H. Cortical reorganisation and chronic pain: implications for rehabilitation. J Rehabil Med 2003;41(Suppl):66–72.

145. Côté P, Hogg-Johnson S, Cassidy JD, et al. Initial patterns of clinical care and recovery from whiplash injuries: a population-based cohort study. Arch Intern Med 2005;165(19): 2257–63.

146. Côté P, Hogg-Johnson S, Cassidy JD, et al. Early aggressive care and delayed recovery from whiplash: isolated finding or reproducible result? Arthritis Rheum 2007;57(5): 861–8.

147. Andersen JC. Stretching before and after exercise: effect on muscle soreness and injury risk. J Athletic Train 2005;40(3):218–20.

148. Herbert RD, de Noronha M, Kamper SJ. Stretching to prevent or reduce muscle soreness after exercise. Cochrane Database Syst Rev 2011;7:CD004577.

149. Grunnesjö MI, Bogefeldt JP, Blomberg SI, et al. A randomized controlled trial of the effects of muscle stretching, manual therapy and steroid injections in addition to "stay active" care

on health-related quality of life in acute or subacute low back pain. Clin Rehabil 2011; 25(11):999–1010.

150. Lee BG, Cho NS, Rhee YG. Effect of two rehabilitation protocols on range of motion and healing rates after arthroscopic rotator cuff repair: aggressive versus limited early passive exercises. Arthroscopy 2012;28(1):34–42.

151. Kay TM, Gross A, Goldsmith CH, et al. Exercises for mechanical neck disorders. Cochrane Database Syst Rev 2005;3:CD004250.

152. Posadzki P, Ernst E, Terry R, et al. Is yoga effective for pain? A systematic review of randomized clinical trials. Complement Ther Med 2011;19(5):281–7.

153. Posadzki P, Ernst E. Yoga for low back pain: a systematic review of randomized clinical trials. Clin Rheumatol 2011;30(9):1257–62.

154. Chuntharapat S, Petpichetchian W, Hatthakit U. Yoga during pregnancy: effects on maternal comfort, labor pain and birth outcomes. Complement Ther Clin Pract 2008;14(2):105–15.

155. Garfinkel MS, Schumacher HR Jr, Husain A, et al. Evaluation of a yoga based regimen for treatment of osteoarthritis of the hands. J Rheumatol 1994;21(12):2341–3.

156. John PJ, Sharma N, Sharma CM, et al. Effectiveness of yoga therapy in the treatment of migraine without aura: a randomized controlled trial. Headache 2007;47(5):654–61.

157. Garfinkel MS, Singhal A, Katz WA, et al. Yoga-based intervention for carpal tunnel syndrome: a randomized trial. J Am Med Assoc 1998;280(18):1601–3.

158. Kuttner L, Chambers CT, Hardial J, et al. A randomized trial of yoga for adolescents with irritable bowel syndrome. Pain Res Manag 2006;11(4):217–23.

159. Williams K, Abildso C, Steinberg L, et al. Evaluation of the effectiveness and efficacy of Iyengar yoga therapy on chronic low back pain. Spine 2009;34(19):2066–76.

160. Sherman KJ, Cherkin DC, Erro J, et al. Comparing yoga, exercise, and a self-care book for chronic low back pain: a randomized, controlled trial. Ann Intern Med 2005;143(12): 849–56.

161. Pushpika Attanayake AM, Somarathna KI, Vyas GH, Dash SC. Clinical evaluation of selected Yogic procedures in individuals with low back pain. Ayu 2010;31(2):245–50.

162. Saper RB, Sherman KJ, Cullum-Duggan D, et al. Yoga for chronic low back pain in a predominantly minority population: a pilot randomized controlled trial. Altern Ther Health Med 2009;15(6):18–27.

163. Sherman KJ, Cherkin DC, Wellman RD, et al. A randomized trial comparing yoga, stretching, and a self-care book for chronic low back pain. Arch Intern Med 2011;171(22): 2019–26.

164. Tilbrook HE, Cox H, Hewitt CE, et al. Yoga for chronic low back pain: a randomized trial. Ann Intern Med 2011;155(9):569–78.

165. Ylinen J, Kautiainen H, Wirén K, et al. Stretching exercises vs manual therapy in treatment of chronic neck pain: a randomized, controlled cross-over trial. J Rehabil Med 2007;39(2): 126–32.

166. Marangoni AH. Effects of intermittent stretching exercises at work on musculoskeletal pain associated with the use of a personal computer and the influence of media on outcomes. Work 2010;36(1):27–37.

167. Ylinen JJ, Takala EP, Nykänen MJ, et al. Effects of twelve-month strength training subsequent to twelve-month stretching exercise in treatment of chronic neck pain. J Strength Cond Res 2006;20(2):304–8.

168. Salo PK, Häkkinen AH, Kautiainen H, et al. Effect of neck strength training on health-related quality of life in females with chronic neck pain: a randomized controlled 1-year follow-up study. Health Qual Life Outcomes 2010;8:48.

169. Häkkinen A, Salo P, Tarvainen U, et al. Effect of manual therapy and stretching on neck muscle strength and mobility in chronic neck pain. J Rehabil Med 2007;39(7):575–9.

170. Häkkinen A, Kautiainen H, Hannonen P, et al. Strength training and stretching versus stretching only in the treatment of patients with chronic neck pain: a randomized one-year follow-up study. Clin Rehabil 2008;22(7):592–600.

171. Ma C, Wu S, Li G, et al. Comparison of miniscalpel-needle release, acupuncture needling, and stretching exercise to trigger point in myofascial pain syndrome. Clin J Pain 2010;26(3): 251–7.
172. Edwards J, Knowles N. Superficial dry needling and active stretching in the treatment of myofascial pain: a randomised controlled trial. Acupunct Med 2003;21(3):80–6.
173. Katalinic OM, Harvey LA, Herbert RD, et al. Stretch for the treatment and prevention of contractures. Cochrane Database Syst Rev 2010;9:CD007455.

CHAPTER 10

Stretch-tolerance Model

In clinic we may sometimes find that yoga and martial arts practitioners who are "stretch experienced" may be less concerned about painful stretching positions than those who are "stretch naïve". This difference in attitude is the basis of the stretch-tolerance model. This model proposes that flexibility training has a psychological desensitizing influence, in which the individual becomes more familiar, less fearful and therefore more tolerant of stretching discomfort/pain.[1,2] In the last decade the stretch-tolerance model has gained popularity and has been used to explain gains in flexibility following acute bouts of stretching and regular stretching, and to explain range of movement (ROM) differences between stiff and flexible individuals.[3-14]

A stretch-tolerance model suggests a learning process in which the individual dissociates pain from injury. Studies on conscious humans apply tensional forces that are well within tolerable pain levels. These forces are probably within safe, non-damaging ranges. Hence, the individual quickly learns that within the tolerable ranges there are no negative consequences to the stretch-pain experience (except for an occasional mild delayed onset muscle soreness (DOMS)).[15] The stretch-tolerance model is in contrast to the previously held assumptions that ROM gains after stretching are the result of adaptive tissue changes.[16] Although there is substantial support for the stretch-tolerance model it raises several paradoxes which will be discussed in this chapter.

This chapter will aim to answer the following questions:

- Can this model explain ROM loss and recovery?
- Does it have any implications for ROM management?
- Does it have any implications for flexibility training?

ORIGIN OF STRETCH-TOLERANCE MODEL

As discussed in Chapter 6, an acute bout of stretching is associated with a transient increase in tissue compliance (or reduced stiffness). This means that the joint can be stretched further using the same level of force (creep deformation). This change in stiffness would be expressed as a right shift in the force–elongation curve (Fig. 10.1). However, these viscoelastic responses are transient, lasting several minutes to an hour (Ch. 6).[9] It has been assumed that regular stretching has a cumulative effect in which this right shift would become permanent, i.e. the tissue would undergo lasting changes becoming longer and more compliant.

Contrary to this expectation, numerous studies demonstrated that the force–elongation profile at the onset of training remained unchanged following several weeks of stretching.[5–14] A right shift was not evident following regular stretching; all that happened was that the point at which a person experienced discomfort shifted to a point further along the force–elongation curve (Fig. 10.2). These findings led to the current view that the increase in ROM is a psychological–sensory phenomenon rather than an adaptive tissue change. However, several other studies using similar testing methods have suggested that regular stretching does bring about adaptive tissue changes.[16–19] So is there a reason why there is such disparity in views in studies that use similar methods?

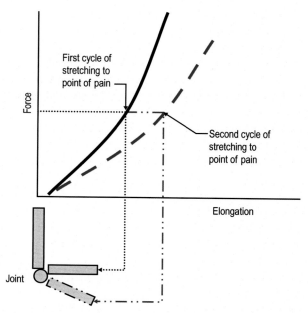

FIGURE 10.1 Range of movement increases owing to a change in tissue stiffness.

STIFF VERSUS LONG

In normal joints a long-term increase in ROM can come about either by an adaptive reduction in the stiffness of the tissues or by an increase in their length, i.e. making the spring softer or longer. Many of the studies that support the stretch-tolerance model measured stiffness, not length (the force–elongation curve is a measure of muscle–tendon stiffness, not length). They are different measures. For example, a 1- metre rope has the same stiffness profile as a 2-metre rope, but of course they are not the same length. An alternative explanation to the stretch-tolerance model is that stiffness remains unchanged but now the muscle is longer. As a consequence the interval between pain and damage has shifted up along the curve, hence the shift in pain experience to a new tension point (Fig. 10.2). It could be argued, therefore, that the stretch-tolerance studies have demonstrated length adaptation, but instead have been interpreted as a pain tolerance phenomenon.

Is it possible for a muscle to undergo adaptive length change while maintaining the same stiffness? As discussed previously, paired muscle groups strive to reach a functional equilibrium at new angles of immobilization or habitual

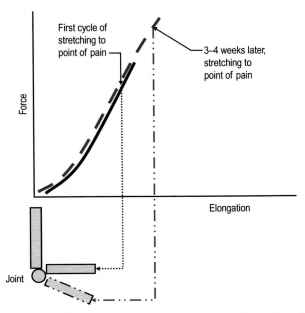

FIGURE 10.2 Range of movement increase as a shift along the force–elongation curve.

use (Ch. 4).[20-22] At these angles they have to achieve optimal force production while maintaining their passive mechanical properties. Such adaptive reorganization has been demonstrated in several animal studies. In one study, immobilization of the muscle in the lengthened position resulted in a 19% increase in the number of sarcomeres in series.[23] Yet there was no significant difference in the stiffness profile between the longer muscle and the control limb (Fig. 10.3). In other words, the normal muscles of the control limb displayed the same stiffness characteristics as the longer (immobilized) muscle.[23] In one study, the animals were still able to maintain isometric contractions of the muscles pertaining to the immobilized joint.[24] It was found that after several weeks the stiffness properties of the muscles returned to values similar to those of normal muscles, although these muscles had undergone adaptive length changes.

Further evidence supporting length versus stiffness differences comes from studies on elderly women and patients with diabetes mellitus and peripheral neuropathy. It was found that older women and patients with these conditions had an ankle stiffness profile similar to the control group. However, the older women and the patient group had a reduced ankle ROM, suggesting "shorter" rather than "stiffer" plantar flexor muscles.[25,26]

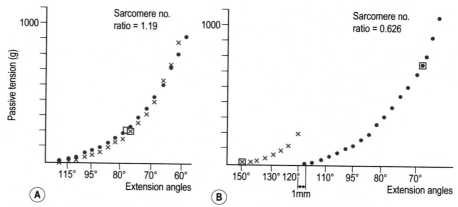

FIGURE 10.3 Force–elongation curve for muscles immobilized in lengthened (A) and shortened (B) positions. X = immobilized muscle and (•) = control limb. In the lengthened position there is an increase in sarcomere ratio yet the stiffness profile is very similar to the control. In B, there is a reduced ratio of serial sarcomeres with a left shift on the curve, implying increased muscle stiffness. *Reprinted from Tabary JC, Tabary C, Tardieu C, et al. Physiological and structural changes in the cat's soleus muscle due to immobilization at different lengths by plaster casts. J Physiol 1972;224(1):231–44, with permission from John Wiley & Sons.*

IS A TOLERANCE MODEL LOGICAL?

Although the tolerance model is well supported by research it creates paradoxes which question its validity or clinical usefulness.

The place to start looking at these contradictions is the relationship between stretching pain and tissue damage – the pain–damage interval. Presumably, the pain associated with stretching is the body's signal that elongation is approximating the upper limits of the tissue's tensile strength. For this reason, high-force, acute bouts of stretching can result in a mild form of DOMS.[15] Assuming that no extensibility or length adaptation has taken place following stretching, the first question is why would our body switch off this protective system after a few weeks of stretching; wouldn't subsequent stretching to a new angle exceed these original dangerous end-limits?

Let us for a minute accept the stretch-tolerance model and perform a hypothetical experiment. Thirty years ago I trained to perform full splits as part of my yoga practice. It took about 2 years of daily training to achieve this yoga posture. However, this agility was completely lost several months after the cessation of stretching. Currently, I have become inflexible to the point that during forward bending I can hardly reach beyond my knees. According to the stretch-tolerance model the flexibility gains of 30 years ago and my current state of inflexibility are the result of stretch tolerance, unrelated to adaptive tissue changes. If this model is correct, I could be anaesthetized from the waist down and perform a full split, at present, without any re-training and without any muscle damage. Furthermore, using the same reasoning and with a dose of anaesthetic, I should have been able to perform a full split, again without any tissue damage, 30 years ago before I even trained for this posture.

Some researchers have also proposed that ROM differences between flexible and stiff individuals are largely the result of their stretch-tolerance differences rather than tissue differences. In two studies that support the stretch-tolerance model it was found that hypermobile women and flexible individuals have greater ROM than their less agile controls, as would be expected.[27,28] However, there was no difference in muscle stiffness between the groups, i.e. no right shift on the force–elongation curve. From these findings the researchers drew the conclusion that the observed differences were due to stretch-tolerance differences rather than physical tissue differences. Re-phrased, they suggest that pain-tolerant individuals are more flexible than pain-"intolerant" individuals. These conclusions can be explored with the same hypothetical exercise used above. Take a group of individuals of similar size and build, and of varying flexibility. Anaesthetize and stretch them to angles which are likely to cause tissue damage. According to the stretch-tolerance model their muscles should fail uniformly at exactly the same angle (since the only difference between individuals is their conscious tolerance of pain, not muscle length or stiffness).

How likely is that? A more reasonable conclusion is that in normal individuals (passive) flexibility is determined by tissue resistance. This will influence the angle at which the person will experience pain and discomfort. This angle will be engaged earlier in individuals with shorter and stiffer tissues. How far a person will stretch beyond that point will depend on their stretch tolerance.

Another paradox of this model is related to the associative nature of stretch tolerance and the extinction of tolerance. It is known that the ROM gains of stretching are lost very rapidly after termination of regular stretching. For example, a break of 4 weeks completely abolishes the ROM gains of 6 weeks of stretching.[29] From a stretch-tolerance perspective it would mean that the associative learning achieved during the 6 weeks of training becomes extinct within 4 weeks of terminating the stretch training. Although such "forgetting" is possible, it is unlikely to occur within a relatively short break of 4 weeks. The fluctuation in ROM in relation to training is more reminiscent of tissue adaption. This was demonstrated in one of the studies that have shown ROM increases and adaptive tissue changes following intensive stretching programme. Re-testing a month after cessation of stretching demonstrated a partial loss of some of these tissue and ROM gains (suggesting a return to the default functional setting; see competition in adaptation, Ch. 12).[17]

The stretch-tolerance model also implies that regular, long-term stretching is the only form of training/physical behaviour that fails to bring about any adaptive tissue changes. Are we comfortable with this notion?

STRETCH-TOLERANCE RELEVANCE TO ROM REHABILITATION

The stretch-tolerance model can be useful clinically in informing us about ROM management in conditions where sensitization may be evident (Ch. 9). However, in conditions where adaptive ROM losses are present this model can be problematic.

Let us apply the anaesthetic experiment clinically. Now imagine a patient with a frozen shoulder who presents with glenohumeral contractures. Is the recovery of ROM the result of a change in stretch tolerance or the result of adaptive elongation? If recovery is all about stretch tolerance we should be able to repeat the experiment suggested above: anaesthetize the glenohumeral joint and stretch it to the anatomical end-range in one go. Although this may seem like a cruel experiment, manipulation under anaesthetic is a common medical procedure to improve ROM in a frozen shoulder. However, the consequence is a catastrophic plastic recovery of ROM in which every tissue in the shoulder is damaged (the "undesirable" plastic elongation, Ch. 6). The list of damage is long: superior, anterior, posterior capsule ruptured, labrum tears, partial tears of the subscapularis tendon, anterior labral detachments and tears of the middle glenohumeral ligament.[30] Hence, applying a tolerance model clinically in conditions where ROM losses are associated with adaptive tissue changes can have disastrous treatment consequences. However, this does not exclude the possibility of concurrent tissue shortening with sensitization and the stretch-tolerance phenomenon (Ch. 9).

IMPLICATION FOR AGILITY TRAINING

The tolerance model can explain some of the ROM gains seen in normal healthy individuals who participate in short-term stretching programmes. However, it cannot explain the profound ROM increases seen in individuals who train regularly for many years. Furthermore, it is unclear how a stretch-tolerance model can inform training practices for individuals who aim to increase their agility, such as in yoga, dance, martial arts or athletic activities that require flexibility. Far more important to flexibility training is an adaptive–behavioural model that includes specificity, overloading and repetition principles.

SUMMARY

- Stretch tolerance is a "learned dissociation" between the experience of stretching pain and injury
- Immediate and short-term ROM gains may be associated with an increase in stretch tolerance
- ROM gains following long-term regular stretching may be associated with stretch tolerance but also with adaptive tissue changes
- A stretch-tolerance model fails to explain ROM loss or recovery in conditions where adaptive tissue changes have taken place
- The stretch-tolerance model is important in conditions in which ROM losses are associated with sensitization (Ch. 9)
- A stretch-tolerance model fails to elucidate the mechanisms underlying long-term gain of flexibility by regular stretch training
- The stretch-tolerance model has no training implications for healthy individuals who aim to increase their agility
- Adaptive–behavioural models are far more informative for agility training and managing recovery in conditions where ROM losses are associated with adaptive tissue changes

REFERENCES

1. Magnusson SP. Passive properties of human skeletal muscle during stretch maneuvers. A review. Scand J Med Sci Sports 1998;8(2):65–77.

2. Magnusson SP, Simonsen EB, Aagaard P, et al. Determinants of musculoskeletal flexability: viscoelastic properties, cross-sectional area, EMG and stretch tolerance. Scand J Med Sci Sports 1997;7:195–202.

3. Zakas A, Balaska P, Grammatikopoulou MG, et al. Acute effects of stretching duration on the range of motion of elderly women. J Bodyw Mov Ther 2005;9:270–6.

4. Whatman C, Knappstein A, Hume P. Acute changes in passive stiffness and range of motion post-stretching. Phys Ther Sport 2006;7:195–200.

5. Mitchell UH, Myrer JW, Hopkins JT, et al. Acute stretch perception alteration contributes to the success of the PNF "contract–relax" stretch. J Sport Rehabil 2007;16(2):85–92.

6. Halbertsma JP, Mulder I, Göeken LN, et al. Repeated passive stretching: acute effect on the passive muscle moment and extensibility of short hamstrings. Arch Phys Med Rehabil 1999;80(4):407–14.

7. Halbertsma JP, van Bolhuis AI, Göeken LN. Sport stretching: effect on passive muscle stiffness of short hamstrings. Arch Phys Med Rehabil 1996;77(7):688–92.

8. Björklund M, Hamberg J, Crenshaw AG. Sensory adaptation after a 2-week stretching regimen of the rectus femoris muscle. Arch Phys Med Rehabil 2001;82:1245–50.

9. LaRoche DP, Connolly DAJ. Effects of stretching on passive muscle tension and response to eccentric exercise. Am J Sports Med 2006;34(6):1000–7.

10. Chan SP, Hong Y, Robinson PD. Flexibility and passive resistance of the hamstrings of young adults using two different static stretching protocols. Scand J Med Sci Sports 2001;11: 81–6.

11. Kubo K, Kanehisa H, Fukunaga T. Effect of stretching training on the viscoelastic properties of human tendon structures in vivo. J Appl Physiol 2002;92:595–601.

12. Folpp H, Deall S, Harvey LA, et al. Can apparent increases in muscle extensibility with regular stretch be explained by changes in tolerance to stretch? Aust J Physiother 2006;52:45–50.

13. Law RY, Harvey LA, Nicholas MK, et al. Stretch exercises increase tolerance to stretch in patients with chronic musculoskeletal pain: a randomized controlled trial. Phys Ther 2009;89(10): 1016–26.

14. Ben M, Harvey LA. Regular stretch does not increase muscle extensibility: a randomized controlled trial. Scand J Med Sci Sports 2010;20(1):136–44.

15. Smith LL, Brunetz MH, Chenier TC, et al. The effects of static and ballistic stretching on delayed onset muscle soreness and creatine kinase. Res Q Exerc Sport 1993;64:103–7.

16. Gajdosik RL. Effects of static stretching on the maximal length and resistance to passive stretch of short hamstring muscles. J Orthop Sports Phys Ther 1991;14(6):250–5.

17. Guissard N, Duchateau J. Effect of static stretch training on neural and mechanical properties of the human plantar-flexor muscles. Muscle Nerve 2004;29(2):248–55.

18. Gajdosik RL, van der Linden DW, McNair PJ, et al. Effects of an eight-week stretching program on the passive-elastic properties and function of the calf muscles of older women. Clin Biomech 2005;20(9):973–83.

19. Reid DA, McNair PJ. Passive force, angle, and stiffness changes after stretching of hamstring muscles. Med Sci Sports Exerc 2004;36(11):1944–8.

20. Aquino CF, Fonseca ST, Gonçalves GG, et al. Stretching versus strength training in lengthened position in subjects with tight hamstring muscles: a randomized controlled trial. Man Ther 2010;15(1):26–31.

21. Scott AB. Change of eye muscle sarcomeres according to eye position. J Pediatr Ophthalmol Strabismus 1994;31(2):85–8.

22. Williams PE, Goldspink G. Changes in sarcomere length and physiological properties in immobilized muscle. J Anat 1978;127(3):459–68.

23. Tabary JC, Tabary C, Tardieu C, et al. Physiological and structural changes in the cat's soleus muscle due to immobilization at different lengths by plaster casts. J Physiol 1972;224(1):231–44.

24. Trudel G, Uhthoff HK. Contractures secondary to immobility: is the restriction articular or muscular? An experimental longitudinal study in the rat knee. Arch Phys Med Rehabil 2000;81(1):6–13.

25. Salsich GB, Mueller MJ, Sahrmann SA. Passive ankle stiffness in subjects with diabetes and peripheral neuropathy versus an age-matched comparison group. Phys Ther 2000;80(4):352–62.

26. Gajdosik RL, van der Linden DW, Williams AK. Influence of age on length and passive elastic stiffness characteristics of the calf muscle–tendon unit of women. Phys Ther 1999;79(9):827–38.

27. Halbertsma JP, Göeken LN. Stretching exercises: effect on passive extensibility and stiffness in short hamstrings of healthy subjects. Arch Phys Med Rehabil 1994;75(9):976–81.

28. Magnusson SP, Julsgaard C, Aagaard P, et al. Viscoelastic properties and flexibility of the human muscle–tendon unit in benign joint hypermobility syndrome. J Rheumatol 2001;28(12):2720–5.

29. Willy RW, Kyle BA, Moore SA, et al. Effect of cessation and resumption of static hamstring muscle stretching on joint range of motion. Orthop Sports Phys Ther 2001;31(3):138–44.

30. Loew M, Heichel TO, Lehner B. Intraarticular lesions in primary frozen shoulder after manipulation under general anesthesia. J Shoulder Elbow Surg 2005;14(1):16–21.

CHAPTER 11

Psychological and Behavioural Considerations in ROM Rehabilitation

A dancer presented in my clinic complaining of severe shoulder range of movement (ROM) limitation and pain. He was previously diagnosed as having "joint damage". He consequently became fearful of re-injury and withdrew from activities which challenged the full shoulder ranges. However, on examination it emerged that his condition was likely to be the stiff phase of frozen shoulder. It was explained to him that frozen shoulder, although a painful condition, is not associated with damage; the joint and its tissues are fully intact, shortened/thickened and sensitive. In the following session, a week later, the patient demonstrated a dramatic increase in shoulder ROM. He explained that once he realized that movement would not damage the joint he could tolerate the discomfort and used the arm in full range during the daily activities.

This example serves to highlight that movement limitations can be self-imposed by beliefs and anxieties associated with injury and pain. These psychological and cognitive factors can be as ROM limiting as physical or neurological impediments (Fig. 11.1). Sometimes treatments that successfully restore the physical limitations of ROM may fail to improve functional activities unless these anxieties are addressed.

This chapter will explore the following topics:

- Can ROM limitations have psychological–behavioural origins?
- Could psychological factors influence ROM recovery?
- How can we reassure the patient that end-range movement is OK?

ACTIVITY AVOIDANCE AS ROM LIMITATION

The patient described above is probably no different from other individuals who have been injured or are in pain. There is a natural fear that movement may cause re-damage or increase the pain intensity.[1] As a consequence, individuals may avoid certain ranges of movement and withdraw from activities which they believe will be painful or harmful.[2-10] Such self-imposed

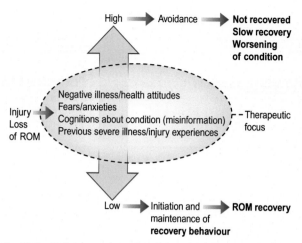

FIGURE 11.1 Psychological and cognitive factors and previous illness experiences can impede the recovery behaviour. ROM, range of movement.

limitations can be seen in spinal conditions as reduced trunk ROM, restricted overhead use of the arm in shoulder conditions and reduced stride length in lower limb conditions. This behaviour would have a negative impact on ROM recovery. It would sustain the dysfunctional motor and tissue adaptation associated with the ROM loss (Ch. 4).[11-14] In contrast, behaviour that frequently challenges movement to the full is essential for recovery. Habitual use of the body drives the positive adaptive processes that underlie ROM normalization (Ch. 4).

Activity avoidance can arise from several factors (Table 11.1):[15] negative beliefs about the condition resulting from inaccurate, misleading or conflicting information from individuals with similar conditions, various health-care practitioners and the media. Activity avoidance can also come about through the experience of pain during specific activities, forming a learned association between pain and movement.[15] This association may be transferred to movement ranges or tasks which are neither harmful nor painful.[7] For example, patients who recover from back pain tend to maintain a restricted movement strategy even when they are pain-free.[7]

Psychological factors that predate the patient's condition could also contribute to avoidance behaviour. Individuals who are naturally anxious may transfer their fears and avoidance behaviour to their current condition.[15] This phenomenon was demonstrated in a large population study on whiplash injury.[16,17] Individuals who exhibit more fear avoidance, who were anxious and depressed and those who had negative illness behaviour *pre-injury* tended to increase their reporting of a whiplash injury, experience more pain and were more

Table 11.1 Characteristics of subclassification of patients with problematic fear-avoidance beliefs

Element	Misinformed avoiders	Learned pain avoiders	Affective avoiders
Emotions	Discouraged	Discouraged	Fearful and highly distressed
Beliefs	Pain indicates harm, and the spine is vulnerable	Pain is benign; spine is sound; and pain should be avoided	Distorted significance of pain and concerns about conditions of the spine
Basis of beliefs	Past experiences with back pain. Information from multiple sources	Inherent value of pain versus function	Emotionally charged misinterpretation of medical information
Behaviours	Hypervigilant but usually willing to perform painful activities in a limited way	Choose to stop activities when they are painful	Profound pain inhibition for movements. Will not attempt activities that might induce pain
Disability	Mild to moderate	Mild to moderate	Severe
Co-morbidities	Uncommon	Uncommon	Catastrophizing, anxiety, depression, concurrent musculoskeletal complaints
Treatment	Information and experiences (exercise) that challenge beliefs about the importance of pain and restore confidence in the spine	Unknown (exercises that desensitize the pain response to physical stimuli might be considered)	Address dysfunctional cognitions and catastrophic thinking. Disconfirm fears through gradual exposure to feared activities

Modified and reprinted from: Rainville J, Smeets RJ, Bendix T, et al. Fear-avoidance beliefs and pain avoidance in low back pain: translating research into clinical practice. Spine J 2011;11(9):895–903, with permission from Elsevier.

likely to receive disability support.[16-18] Similarly, the development of serious back pain disability can be predicted more accurately from the psychosocial history of the individual than from structural/degenerative changes in the spine.[19]

The cognitions and anxieties about movement may feed a widening gap between an assumed incapacity and the current "potential" physical capacity (Fig. 11.2). For example, in patients with acute low back pain, pain-related fears and catastrophizing can be more indicative of their physical ability to lift than pain intensity itself.[20] This gap tends to widen with conditions of longer duration or greater intensity.[12,13,21,22] Hence, an important component of ROM management is to narrow this gap by redefining and exploring with the patient what degree of loss is assumed and what is real; and this can sometimes be difficult to establish.

REASSURANCE

It was demonstrated in patients with chronic back conditions that pain and functionality can improve as much with cognitive–behavioural approaches as

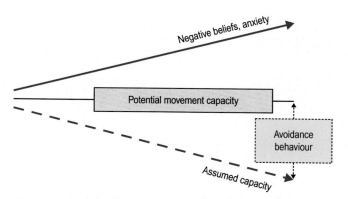

FIGURE 11.2 Cognitions and anxieties about the condition may feed the avoidance behaviour, widening the gap between the assumed and potential physical capacity. This gap can be reduced by cognitive and behavioural interventions.

with physical exercise.[23,24] It seems that both treatment modalities share a similar underlying process for improvement. They both convey a message to the patient that movement is OK, alleviating the anxiety/fear/catastrophizing associated with the condition.[23,25,26] Reassurance can have a profound influence on recovery. Cognitive, psychological and behavioural transformations can help to reduce pain, improve movement capacity, facilitate a return to more normal occupational and recreational activities and reduce health-seeking behaviour.[23,27–33]

Reassurance can be provided in different forms depending on the factors that underlie the avoidance behaviour. Cognition-related avoidance can be managed by providing the patient with information about the condition.[15] Experience-related avoidance can be alleviated by a gradual reintroduction of tasks and movement ranges from which the patient withdrew (graded exposure), as well as cognitive reassurance.[15,34] Patients who exhibit affective, anxiety-related avoidance may partly respond to behavioural forms of reassurance but may not respond well to reasoning or cognitive reassurance. These patients may benefit from psychological counselling as part of their overall management.[15]

Cognition and behaviour are inseparable – a change in cognitions about the condition will influence the person's recovery behaviour. Equally, challenging behaviour by introducing non-aggravating movement experiences can influence how a person perceives their condition and embolden them to experiment with movement which they fear (Fig. 11.3).[35] Hence, reassurance can be provided cognitively or behaviourally, but usually it is a mixture of both.

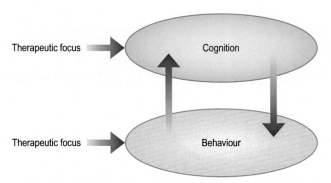

FIGURE 11.3 Reassurance can be provided cognitively and/or behaviourally. A change in cognition can bring about a change in behaviour, and equally challenging movement behaviour can bring about a change in condition-related cognitions.

Cognitive reassurance

When an individual experiences pain or movement limitation they create a personal story about their condition. This internal narrative is derived from numerous sources and previous experiences. It often contains negative messages that are mixed with anxiety and catastrophic thoughts ("shoulder is damaged, seen torn capsules on the internet, a friend had surgery and was unable to play tennis again, will I ever be able to return to playing tennis?"…). An important part of management is to help the patient turn negative narratives into positive ones.

There are several ways in which patients can be helped to transform their cognitions/narratives. Providing patients with relevant information about their condition is an important part of this process;[36–38] in particular, information which they can do something about.[39] Individuals who have a better understanding of their condition are more likely to take up activities that challenge their losses. For example, the patient with the frozen shoulder was given information that emphasized the positive aspect of the condition – that it was self-limiting and unlikely to result in any disability. There was an emphasis on describing the mechanism associated with tissue adaptation and how this process could be facilitated by their behaviour and daily activities. There was also a detailed explanation of the difference between the pain of injury and the pain of sensitization – thereby, *dissociating pain from damage*. Using the same approach, patients who have tissue damage underlying their ROM losses can be informed about tissue repair processes and the importance of movement in supporting these processes, rather than focusing on the extent of tissue damage.

Generally, there is little therapeutic value – and potentially even a negative effect – in using anatomical and biomechanical models for pain or diagnosis that do not support return to function.[40] Patients' fears and anxieties may be increased by a detailed description of underlying damage, and use of terms such as "deterioration" or "degeneration". This may be partly due to the disempowering nature of this form of information which focuses on factors that are outside the patient's control.

Focusing on the "abled self" rather than the "disabled self" can also be part of reassurance – pointing out to patients what they can do, rather than what they cannot do. For example, patients with chronic back pain can be virtually symptom-free during demanding physical activities such as gardening, playing football or even windsurfing. This would be pointed out during the session, focusing on these "abled" activities.

Behavioural reassurance

Behavioural reassurance aims to provide movement experiments in which the patient can reassess what is real and assumed loss. A useful clinical tool to reinforce such positive messages is the graded challenge described in Chapter 6. These movement challenges are performed mostly within pain-free, comfortable ranges, amplifying the four task parameters. It is hoped that through these positive experiences the individual will learn to dissociate movement from pain and injury.

Beyond the session the behavioural reassurance aims to gradually expose the patient to the activities which they fear and avoid.[29–31,41,42] The patient can be invited to make a wish-list of exercise or activities, in order of importance to them. If, for example, the chosen exercise is to return to tennis after shoulder surgery, this would be set as one of the therapeutic goals. The graded challenge can start with serving a tennis ball against a wall for, say, 5 minutes a day, with the serving position below shoulder height. The range parameter can be challenged by incrementally raising the tennis stroke towards shoulder height and gradually above it. The force parameter can be increased by standing further away from the wall, say, doubling the distance. The velocity parameter can be gradually increased by performing the movement faster and endurance by increasing the duration/repetition of strokes. It is important to consult and involve the patient in developing the graded challenge, including the scheduling of the exposure and the setting of short- and long-term goals and time scales for the return to activity.[43]

Reassurance for the therapist

A common clinical concern for the therapist is the safety of the ROM challenge, i.e. the therapist's anxieties may also create a clinical gap between the real and assumed loss. This is partly associated with assessment and diagnostic uncertainties. Even a simple test such as ROM examination can be misleading. It is often affected by the patient's fear of pain/re-injury, or from the simple fact that physical examinations can be low on either validity or reliability.[44–52] Hence, the actual level of damage can remain undetermined and there is always the possibility that the patient's fears may represent real, safety-related limitations. There is added uncertainty as to how the patient will respond to the treatment. These uncertainties could erode the therapist's own confidence in the safety of the treatment and negatively influence management. It could also feed into the patient's negative beliefs and avoidance behaviour.[53] So therapists also need reassurance.

The solution to this conundrum is not easily achieved during examination. It can be partly determined by understanding pain and tissue repair processes, as was discussed in Chapter 9. However, there is always the niggling thought that we may have missed something during the assessment. Another solution is to accept that uncertainty and plan a management programme within a graded challenge model. With this form of clinical management the physical capacity of the patient can be safely established during the behavioural experiment.

Clinical note – in my clinical experience graded challenge has been an invaluable therapeutic tool. Over the years I have managed to help patients return to various activities which they (and I) never imagined they could do again.

ROM LOSS AND PSYCHOLOGICAL DISTRESS

As a consequence of ROM loss and functionality loss, patients often experience feelings such as disappointment, anger, frustration, grief, helplessness and depression. They may feel that their body has let them down. Such physical losses are often also associated with a negative change in body and self-image.[54–56]

The therapeutic relationship can have an important role in alleviating the psychological distress associated with the condition and in supporting the patient to return to functionality.[37,57,58] Clinical attitudes that include being attentive to the patient's emotional state, empathy, being non-judgemental, caring and encouraging should be the bedrock of management.

Working in the psychological dimension and with body image is discussed in more detail in Lederman.[59].

SUMMARY

- ROM loss can be maintained by avoidance behaviour due to fear of pain and re-injury

- Anxieties about movement can be due to misinformation, a learned association between pain and movement or from anxiety traits that predate the condition
- The alleviation of movement-related anxieties can be in the cognitive and behavioural dimensions
- In the cognitive dimension, reassurance can be given by providing information about the condition, in particular positive messages that increase the individual's belief in their ability to care for and control their condition
- Reassurance in the behavioural dimension can include a gradual reintroduction of activities which are important for the patient
- Activities can be introduced using the graded challenge
- ROM losses are often associated with psychological distress and should be acknowledged in the patient's management
- Reassurance – it is all about focusing on the "half-filled glass" …
- What you say can be as important as what you do with the patient

REFERENCES

1. Kori S, Miller R, Todd D. Kinesiophobia: a new view of chronic pain behaviour. Pain Manag 1990;35–43.
2. Poiraudeau S, Rannou F, Baron G, et al. Fear-avoidance beliefs about back pain in patients with subacute low back pain. Pain 2006;124:305–11.
3. Leeuw M, Goossens ME, Linton SJ, et al. The fear-avoidance model of musculoskeletal pain: current state of scientific evidence. J Behav Med 2007;30(1):77–94.
4. Shaw WS, Pransky G, Patterson W, et al. Patient clusters in acute, work-related back pain based on patterns of disability risk factors. J Occup Environ Med 2007;49(2):185–93.
5. Elfving B, Andersson T, Grooten WJ. Low levels of physical activity in back pain patients are associated with high levels of fear-avoidance beliefs and pain catastrophizing. Physiother Res Int 2007;12(1):14–24.
6. Thomas JS, France CR. Pain-related fear is associated with avoidance of spinal motion during recovery from low back pain. Spine 2007;32(16):E460–6.
7. Thomas JS, France CR, Lavender SA, et al. Effects of fear of movement on spine velocity and acceleration after recovery from low back pain. Spine 2008;33(5):564–70.
8. George SZ, Wittmer VT, Fillingim RB, et al. Fear-avoidance beliefs and temporal summation of evoked thermal pain influence self-report of disability in patients with chronic low back pain. J Occup Rehabil 2006;16(1):95–108.
9. Severeijns R, Vlaeyen JW, van den Hout MA, et al. Pain catastrophizing predicts pain intensity, disability, and psychological distress independent of the level of physical impairment. Clin J Pain 2001;17(2):165–72.
10. Woby S, Watson P, Roach N, et al. Adjustment to chronic low back pain: the relative influence of fear-avoidance beliefs, catastrophising, and appraisals of control. Behav Res Ther 2004;42:761–74.
11. Sions JM, Hicks GE. Fear-avoidance beliefs are associated with disability in older American adults with low back pain. Phys Ther 2011;91(4):525–34.
12. Grotle M, Vøllestad NK, Veierød MB, et al. Fear-avoidance beliefs and distress in relation to disability in acute and chronic low back pain. Pain 2004;112(3):343–52.
13. Grotle M, Vøllestad NK, Brox JI. Clinical course and impact of fear-avoidance beliefs in low back pain: prospective cohort study of acute and chronic low back pain: II. Spine 2006;31(9):1038–46.

14. Boersma K, Linton SJ. How does persistent pain develop? An analysis of the relationship between psychological variables, pain and function across stages of chronicity. Behav Res Ther 2005;43(11):1495–507.

15. Rainville J, Smeets RJ, Bendix T, et al. Fear-avoidance beliefs and pain avoidance in low back pain: translating research into clinical practice. Spine J 2011;11(9):895–903.

16. Mykletun A, Glozier N, Wenzel HG, et al. Reverse causality in the association between whiplash and symptoms of anxiety and depression: the HUNT study. Spine 2011;36(17):1380–6.

17. Wenzel HG, Vasseljen O, Mykletun A, et al. Pre-injury health-related factors in relation to self-reported whiplash: longitudinal data from the HUNT study, Norway. Eur Spine J 2012;21(8):1528–35.

18. Kamper SJ, Maher CG, Menezes Costa L, et al. Does fear of movement mediate the relationship between pain intensity and disability in patients following whiplash injury? A prospective longitudinal study. Pain 2012;153(1):113–19.

19. Carragee E, Alamin TF, Miller JL, Carragee JM. Discographic, MRI and psychosocial determinants of low back pain disability and remission: a prospective study in subjects with benign persistent back pain. Spine J 2005;5(1):24–35.

20. Swinkels-Meewisse IE, Roelofs J, Oostendorp RA, et al. Acute low back pain: pain-related fear and pain catastrophizing influence physical performance and perceived disability. Pain 2006;120(1–2):36–43.

21. Pincus T, Vogel S, Burton AK, et al. Fear avoidance and prognosis in back pain: a systematic review and synthesis of current evidence. Arthritis Rheum 2006;54(12):3999–4010.

22. Vangronsveld K, Peters M, Goossens M, et al. The influence of movement and pain catastrophising on daily pain and disability in individuals with acute whiplash injury: a daily diary study. Pain 2008;139:449–57.

23. Smeets RJ, Vlaeyen JW, Kester AD, et al. Reduction of pain catastrophizing mediates the outcome of both physical and cognitive-behavioral treatment in chronic low back pain. J Pain 2006;7(4):261–71.

24. Critchley DJ, Ratcliffe J, Noonan S, et al. Effectiveness and cost-effectiveness of three types of physiotherapy used to reduce chronic low back pain disability: a pragmatic randomized trial with economic evaluation. Spine 2007;32(14):1474–8.

25. Mannion AF, Muntener M, Taimela S, et al. A randomized clinical trial of three active therapies for chronic low back pain. Spine 1999;24:2435–48.

26. Steptoe A, Edwards S, Moses J, et al. The effects of exercise training on mood and perceived coping ability in anxious adults from the general population. J Psychosom Res 1989;33(5):537–47.

27. Skinner JB, Erskine A, Pearce S, et al. The evaluation of a cognitive behavioural treatment programme in outpatients with chronic pain. J Psychosom Res 1990;34(1):13–9.

28. Burton AK, Waddell, G, Tillotson KM, et al. Information and advice to patients with back pain can have a positive effect: a randomised controlled trial of a novel educational booklet in primary care. Spine 1999;24:2484–91.

29. Linton SJ, Ryberg M. A cognitive-behavioral group intervention as prevention for persistent neck and back pain in a non-patient population: a randomized controlled trial. Pain 2001;90(1–2):83–90.

30. Linton SJ, Boersma K, Jansson M, et al. The effects of cognitive-behavioral and physical therapy preventive interventions on pain-related sick leave: a randomized controlled trial. Clin J Pain 2005;21(2):109–19.

31. Linton SJ, Nordin E. A 5-year follow-up evaluation of the health and economic consequences of an early cognitive behavioral intervention for back pain: a randomized, controlled trial. Spine 2006;31(8):853–8.

32. Hoffman BM, Papas RK, Chatkoff DK, et al. Meta-analysis of psychological interventions for chronic low back pain. Health Psychol 2007;26(1):1–9.

33. Williams AC, Richardson PH, Nicholas MK, et al. Inpatient vs. outpatient pain management: results of a randomised controlled trial. Pain 1996;66(1):13–22.

34. Vlaeyen JW, de Jong J, Geilen M, et al. Graded exposure in vivo in the treatment of pain-related fear: a replicated single-case experimental design in four patients with chronic low back pain. Behav Res Ther 2001;39(2):151–66.

35. Vlaeyen JW, Haazen IW, Schuerman JA, et al. Behavioural rehabilitation of chronic low back pain: comparison of an operant treatment, an operant-cognitive treatment and an operant-respondent treatment. Br J Clin Psychol 1995;34:95–118.

36. Burton AK, Waddell G, Tillotson KM, et al. Information and advice to patients with back pain can have a positive effect: a randomised controlled trial of a novel educational booklet in primary care. Spine 1999;24:2484–91.

37. Linton SJ, Andersson T. Can chronic disability be prevented? A randomized trial of a cognitive-behavior intervention and two forms of information for patients with spinal pain. Spine 2000;25(21):2825–31.

38. Moseley GL, Nicholas MK, Hodges PW. A randomized controlled trial of intensive neuro-physiology education in chronic low back pain. Clin J Pain 2004;20(5):324–30.

39. Crow R, Gage H, Hampson S, et al. The role of expectancies in the placebo effect and their use in the delivery of health care: a systematic review. Health Technol Assess 1999;3(3):1–96.

40. Louw A, Diener I, Butler DS, et al. The effect of neuroscience education on pain, disability, anxiety, and stress in chronic musculoskeletal pain. Arch Phys Med Rehabil 2011;92:2041–56.

41. Linton SJ, Boersma K, Jansson M, et al. A randomized controlled trial of exposure in vivo for patients with spinal pain reporting fear of work-related activities. Eur J Pain 2008;12(6):722–30.

42. Vlaeyen JW, Linton SJ. Fear-avoidance model of chronic musculoskeletal pain: 12 years on. Pain 2012;153(6):1144–7.

43. Pfingsten M. Functional restoration: it depends on an adequate mixture of treatment. Schmerz 2001;15(6):492–8.

44. Paulet T, Fryer G. Inter-examiner reliability of palpation for tissue texture abnormality in the thoracic paraspinal region. Int J Osteopath Med 2009;12(3):92–6.

45. May S, Littlewood C, Bishop A. Reliability of procedures used in the physical examination of non-specific low back pain: a systematic review. Aust J Physiother 2006;52(2):91–102.

46. van Trijffel E, Anderegg Q, Bossuyt PM, et al. Inter-examiner reliability of passive assessment of intervertebral motion in the cervical and lumbar spine: a systematic review. Man Ther 2005;10(4):256–69.

47. Seffinger MA, Najm WI, Mishra SI, et al. Reliability of spinal palpation for diagnosis of back and neck pain: a systematic review of the literature. Spine 2004;29(19):E413–25.

48. Dunk NM, Chung YY, Compton DS, et al. The reliability of quantifying upright standing postures as a baseline diagnostic clinical tool. J Manip Physiol Ther 2004;27(2):91–6.

49. Hollerwöger D. Methodological quality and outcomes of studies addressing manual cervical spine examinations: a review. Man Ther 2006;11(2):93–8.

50. McCaw ST, Bates BT. Biomechanical implications of mild leg length inequality. Br J Sports Med 1991;25(1):10–13.

51. Mannello DM. Leg length inequality. J Manip Physiol Ther 1992;15(9):576–90.

52. Levangie PK. Four clinical tests of sacroiliac joint dysfunction: the association of test results with innominate torsion among patients with and without low back pain. Phys Ther 1999;79(11):1043–57.

53. Poiraudeau S, Rannou F, Baron G, et al. Fear-avoidance beliefs about back pain in patients with subacute low back pain. Pain 2006;124:305–11.

54. Moseley GL, Zalucki NM, Wiech K. Tactile discrimination, but not tactile stimulation alone, reduces chronic limb pain. Pain 2008;137(3):600–8.

55. Moseley GL. I can't find it! Distorted body image and tactile dysfunction in patients with chronic back pain. Pain 2008;140(1):239–43.

56. Lotze M, Moseley GL. Role of distorted body image in pain. Curr Rheumatol Rep 2007;9(6):488–96.

57. Lederman T. Touch as a therapeutic intervention. In: Liam T, editor. Morphodynamics of osteopathy. Stuttgart: Hippokrates; 2006.

58. Miciak M, Gross DP, Joyce A. A review of the psychotherapeutic "common factors" model and its application in physical therapy: the need to consider general effects in physical therapy practice. Scand J Caring Sci 2012;26(2):394–403.

59. Lederman E. The science and practice of manual therapy. 2nd ed. Edinburgh: Churchill Livingstone; 2005.

CHAPTER 12

Towards a Functional Approach

This chapter will explore how to integrate the various principles discussed in previous chapters into a unified, functional range of movement (ROM) rehabilitation approach.

The principal aim in ROM rehabilitation is to plan a management that takes into account various patient-related processes. They include the processes underlying the ROM loss, such as the dimension in which the ROM loss occurs – are they related to adaptive tissue changes (tissue dimension), motor control losses or sensitization (neurological dimension), or are they related to fear of movement (psychological dimension)? We also need to consider the patient's ability to execute the recovery behaviour. This will determine the level at which the management is pitched – managed, assisted, functional or extra-functional.

This chapter will explore the following topics:

- How is ROM management matched to the patient's condition?
- When do we use functional or traditional stretching?
- When do we use managed or assisted approaches?
- Do different conditions need specific ROM rehabilitation?
- How can we create a recovery environment beyond the session?

THE POTENCY OF ROM CHALLENGE

Imagine for a moment that ROM rehabilitation is some form of medication rather than a physical procedure. As such, its potency depends of several ingredients which have been identified in the previous chapters: specificity of the challenge (Ch. 5), overloading or amplifying activity at end-range (Ch. 6) and the need for frequent repetition of the ROM challenge (Ch. 7). Added to these is the importance of active versus passive ROM challenges, use of whole rather than fragmented movement and the importance of goal-orientated movement (Ch. 8). ROM management is likely to be more successful when it contains

Table 12.1 The therapeutic potential of various forms of range of movement (ROM) management. Approaches at the top of the table are likely to be more effective than approaches at the bottom. Traditional stretching approaches are within the shaded area. "Yes/no" implies that the challenge may only provide the effective ingredient in certain situations

	Management/ROM challenge	Effective ingredients for ROM adaptation				
		Specificity	Overloading	Repetition	Active	Whole and goal
Functional	Recovery behaviour	Yes	Yes	Yes	Yes	Yes
	Managed recovery behaviour	Yes	Yes	Yes	Yes	Yes
	Assisted recovery behaviour (functional stretching)	Yes	Yes	No	Yes	Yes
Extra-functional	Ballistic stretching	No	Yes/no	No	Yes/no	Yes/no
	Dynamic stretching	No	Yes/no	No	Yes/no	Yes/no
	Muscle energy techniques	No	Yes/no	No	Yes	No
	Passive stretching	No	No	No	No	No
	Spinal manipulation	No	No	No	No	No
	Traction	No	No	No	No	No
	Articulation	No	No	No	No	No
	Harmonic	No	No	No	No	No
	Strain counter-strain	No	No	No	No	No
	Cranial	No	No	No	No	No

the maximum number of these ingredients and less so as their number declines (Table 12.1).

Using this table, ROM challenges can be grouped into functional and extra-functional approaches and their therapeutic efficacy can be evaluated. The recovery behaviour is at the top of this table as it contains the maximum number of ingredients, providing the ideal conditions required for ROM recovery; it is natural, free and works for most people most of the time. It is followed by managed and assisted recovery behaviour (functional stretching). Below the functional approaches are all the traditional stretching techniques. At this point there is also a drop in the number of the effective ingredients, suggesting a decline in therapeutic potential.

This hierarchy of effectiveness can be exemplified in the active stretching approaches, such as muscle energy techniques. They contain only some of the effective ingredients (overloading and active) and are missing others, such as specificity and repetition. The absence of these ingredients is likely to reduce their therapeutic effectiveness in assisting ROM recovery (see Ch. 1). However, more research is required to explore the relationship between the effective ingredients and therapeutic success. In the meantime, this can be resolved by striving to provide the functional ROM management which contains the full set of effective ingredients.

DETERMINING THE LEVEL AND FORM OF ROM REHABILITATION

Assuming that the patient has a condition which is likely to respond to ROM rehabilitation, the next clinical task is to determine the level of ROM rehabilitation: whether it should be functional (managed or assisted) or extra-functional using traditional stretching methods (Fig. 12.1).

Recovery behaviour

All patients should be made aware of the benefits of a functional approach, highlighting the importance of specificity, overloading and repetition, i.e. "whatever you do, do more, to the end-limit and more often". Patients who have the capacity to engage in this behaviour, who are autonomous and who

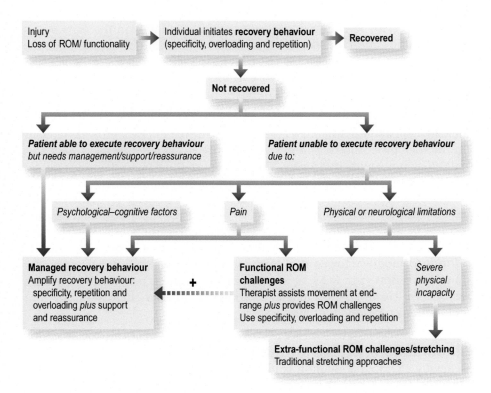

FIGURE 12.1 Clinical reasoning in range of movement (ROM) rehabilitation: determining the level and form of ROM challenges.

have high self-efficacy and who are already challenging their movement ranges may need only this general advice.

Managed recovery behaviour

At a managed level the primary task is to identify daily tasks that provide effective ROM challenges, e.g. for a patient with restricted hip – "do more walking". It may include focusing and amplifying specific task parameters within these daily activities (force, speed, range and endurance) – "do more walking taking wider steps" (range parameter). It could also include rectifying compensatory patterns that result in underloading of the affected joints, e.g. "avoid swinging the leg to the side when walking". Within a managed level we also provide psychological–cognitive reassurance, in particular if the patient's recovery behaviour is impeded by movement-related anxieties – "it might be uncomfortable as you walk but its not causing any damage".

Assisted recovery behaviour

This level is important if the patient is capable of performing whole movement, but unable to provide sufficient overloading to effectively challenge their ROM losses. This level of management would be suitable in the early stages after immobilization or when multiple injuries or co-morbidities impede the recovery behaviour. Under these circumstances the end-range can be reached with assistance by the therapist. Once in this position, the patient is encouraged to "take over" and performs different functional tasks (see graded challenge and the task parameters, Ch. 6, and the accompanying video).

Management at the assisted level can result in the patient becoming dependent on the therapist. Since self-care is essential for ROM rehabilitation such attitudes may impede their recovery. Therefore, once the patient demonstrates an ability to perform the ROM challenge effectively they should rapidly progress to a managed approach. This progression may be difficult for patients who have a tendency for low autonomy or low self-efficacy or who have an external locus of health. They will often steer the treatment towards or wish to remain within an assisted approach. Sometimes this attitude of dependency can be difficult to modify. However, it does not represent a significant drawback in minor and short-term ROM losses. At worst the patient may need a few extra treatments. However, dependency becomes a problem in conditions that require longer treatment durations.

Management at extra-functional level

Generally, ROM rehabilitation at the extra-functional level should be reserved for situations in which the patient has lost their movement capacity to a level at which they are unable to carry out the recovery behaviour or whole movement patterns.

Active approaches can be used when a patient is still able to execute an active movement at a particular joint but not whole functional tasks. Passive ROM challenges are provided in full by the therapist. As such, they will only be useful if the patient is unable to execute any active movement. This clinical scenario is seen in motor control losses and contractures following peripheral and central nervous system damage. However, such losses are often persistent and the therapeutic effects of passive stretching are expected to be very limited.

In summary, classifying the challenges by their effective ingredients suggests a therapeutic hierarchy with functional approaches at the top and extra-functional ones at the bottom. This hierarchy is independent of the causative condition, but is dependent on the individual's movement ability, i.e. *the treatment always seeks to be at a functional level regardless of the cause.*

PROGRESSIVE AND REGRESSIVE MANAGEMENT

A patient has arrived in your clinic complaining of reduced ROM of the hip as a result of a long-term injury. The patient has driven to the clinic, walked in, perhaps having to deal with a few steps on the way. At which level do we start the treatment? Is there any point in treating the patient lying down if they can already walk?

There is no therapeutic value in challenging movement at a level below the patient's capacity. Whenever possible the patient should be treated or trained within their movement capacity. If the patient can stand then rehabilitation of the hip should be in weight-bearing activities. Exercising on the floor or treatment table would be a regressive approach. Below are some considerations for developing a progressive ROM management:

- Avoid extra-functional challenges if the patient is able to perform functional tasks
- Avoid assistance if the patient is able to fully carry out the recovery behaviour
- Avoid fragmentation if the patient is able to perform whole movement
- Avoid a passive approach if the patient is active

Is there a place for a regressive management? It is reasoned that it is easier to train in a recumbent position or to fragment movement and then transfer this experience to more complex functional tasks. Such a training/rehabilitation approach is likely to be ineffective as it is in conflict with specificity and motor control principles (Chs 5 and 8). Another common argument is that regressive management may help to reassure the patient that movement is safe. There may be some merit in this form of reassurance. However, it can also convey the opposite message – that movement is unsafe, especially if the patient is already able to execute more demanding daily activities. Ideally, reassurance in the form of regressive management should be quickly replaced by the reassurance of progressive management.

In summary, ROM management should always be progressive, striving up to the next level (Table 12.1).

THE CONTEXT SHORT-CUT

The specificity principle provides us with a useful planning short-cut: a context principle. This principle allows grouping of the body into areas that can be rehabilitated in a similar manner.

The body can be divided into areas that typify their role during functional movement (Table 12.2): upper and lower limbs, trunk, and head and neck. The upper limbs are associated with reaching–retrieving, carrying, lifting, manipulation of objects, etc. The lower limbs are associated with weight-bearing activities and locomotion. The trunk is more difficult to classify as it plays a part in all movements. We often associate it with bending, twisting, supporting movements of the limbs such as reaching and stationary positions such as sitting. The head and neck are mostly associated with movement related to the senses, following the gaze or a sound, feeding actions and so on. So, at the basic level of movement context, a joint does what a joint does. A hip, knee, ankle and foot all have their distinct patterns of anatomical movement (physiological range). At the next movement level, all the leg joints move in patterns that reflect what the whole leg does, within the context of what the person does with their legs, within the context of their environment, e.g. stand, run, squat,

Table 12.2 The context short-cut in managing range of movement (ROM) recovery. Different body areas have typical roles during shared functional movement. Within each area, the ROM challenges are largely universal regardless of the joint affected. Many daily activities can be exaggerated to challenge ROM losses at home. Challenges are an extension of the area's functional role

Body area	Typical role during shared functional movement	Joints affected	Home ROM challenges
Upper limb	Reaching–retrieving, holding, lifting, manipulating objects, etc.	Shoulder, elbow, wrist and hand	Same as functional role but exaggerated (overloading and amplification)
Lower limb	Walk, stand, step over obstacles, stairs, run, etc.	Hip, knee, ankle and foot	Same as functional role but exaggerated (overloading and amplification)
Trunk	Support all movement, bending, side reaching/bending, twisting, sitting, etc.	Lumbar and dorsal spine	Same as functional role but exaggerated (overloading and amplification)
Head and neck	Follow eye movements and sound, feeding, etc.	Cervical joints	Same as functional role but exaggerated (overloading and amplification)

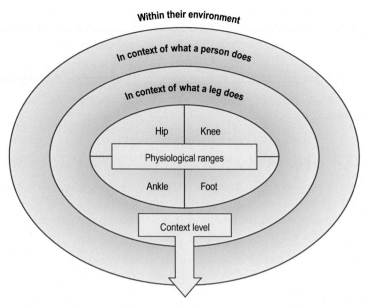

FIGURE 12.2 Context principle in the leg. All lower limb joints have their unique physiological range of movement (ROM). However, at a functional level ROM rehabilitation is similar for all joints.

climb stairs, play tennis (functional context). Hence, any particular area or joint is rehabilitated in the context of what it does functionally (Fig. 12.2).

Now, let us make an obvious observation: what we do with our arms that we do not do with our legs. This means that, for the joints of the upper limb, the rehabilitation will be unique to that body area, and similar to all the area's joints. Reaching, lifting and manipulating objects can be used to challenge ROM losses in the shoulder but also in the elbow. The choice of challenges would be very different for the legs. Here, weight-bearing and locomotion activities can be used to rehabilitate ROM loss in the hip but equally in the knee or ankle. This line of reasoning can be applied to the trunk and neck. Regardless of the location of ROM restriction, a functional task such as sitting and reaching forwards or sideways will challenge the spine as a whole, dorsal and lumbar. Similarly the neck can be challenged with the head leading the movements. For example, rotation ROM can be challenged by holding a book further to the left or right while reading.

There is a further management advantage in a contextual line of reasoning. The movement challenges will be mostly the same for restrictions due to meniscus or anterior cruciate ligament surgery or contractures following immobilization. Regardless of the cause, the knee still has to move within its physiological ranges, which in turn need to be challenged within the context of what the person does with the leg in their environment (get up, walk, play tennis, etc.).

Overall, the context principle promotes management economy. It only requires the awareness of the functional role of the area being rehabilitated rather than having to learn and apply a range of specific exercises for each joint or for different conditions.

CO-CREATING A ROM RECOVERY ENVIRONMENT

All adaptation processes associated with ROM recovery depend on the individual's actions within their environment. ROM rehabilitation should therefore be all-inclusive, multidimensional and addressing the person within their environment (Fig. 12.3).

At the interaction of the person and their environment the patient can be encouraged to identify social, occupational or recreational situations that would increase their exposure to ROM challenges. In the psychological and cognitive dimensions management focuses on alleviating fear, providing information about the condition, which empowers the patient, setting goals and supporting the patient in the journey of recovery.

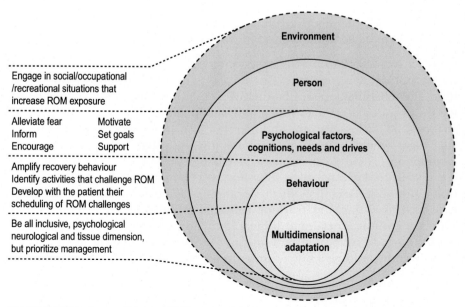

FIGURE 12.3 Co-creating a multidimensional environment for range of movement (ROM) recovery.

In the behavioural dimension the focus is on amplifying the specificity, over-loading and repetition components of the recovery behaviour. Behavioural management also includes engaging the patient in daily activities and ampli-fying them to provide effective ROM challenges. The scheduling of the ROM challenges – how often and for how long – are also within this behavioural sphere.

Prioritizing managment

The general aim of a functional approach is to be all-inclusive, exploring the multidimensional processes associated with the patient's condition. However, management that is all-inclusive can be too complex to execute and can come at the cost of being unfocused and even ineffective. Hence, in clinic, we are often required to prioritize management and focus on particular processes.

Generally, prioritizing works on what process requires most immediate atten-tion: it is about short- and long-term treatment goals. This is exemplified in Fig. 12.4:

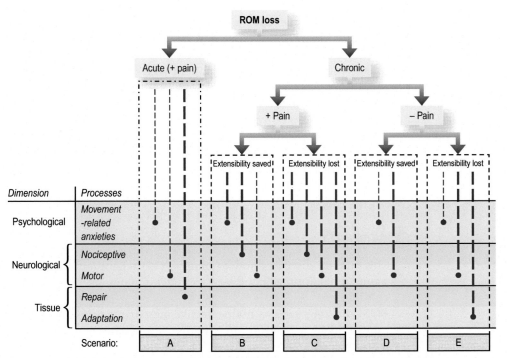

FIGURE 12.4 Prioritizing and minimizing management. Different forms of range of movement (ROM) losses require unique management (dashed lines) and prioritization (heavier dashed lines).

A: Represents an acute injury. Here, the priority is to support repair processes (tissue dimension). In these conditions, rehabilitation of motor control is not urgent and can be added at a later date if active ROM losses are present (neurological dimension). All that is needed is to reassure the patient that movement is beneficial and to maintain daily activities (psychological dimension).

B: In this scenario, ROM losses are chronic and are associated with pain and sensitization, but there are no obvious adaptive tissue changes, for example chronic low back and neck pain. Here, the priority is within the neurological and psychological dimensions, working with nociceptive processes and desensitization as well as with psychological–cognitive and behavioural factors associated with pain experience. Rehabilitation of motor control ROM could wait, but daily activity should be maintained to prevent disuse. In this scenario, ROM challenges directed at tissue processes are unlikely to be therapeutically useful, e.g. passive stretching.

C: In this scenario, the patient presents with ROM loss associated with adaptive tissue shortening and pain, e.g. "fresh" post-surgical contracture. This is probably the most complex management. It often requires working simultaneously in all three dimensions. However, if the pain is moderate to severe, desensitization and pain alleviation may become the treatment priority. The treatment can progress to the tissue dimension (adaptive tissue changes) and neurological dimension (motor control) when pain levels become more tolerable.

D: This example may represent a patient who has active ROM losses, such as muscle weakness, but not associated with adaptive tissue shortening or pain. The treatment priority in this case would be on motor control / neuromuscular recovery (neurological dimension).

E: This scenario is commonly observed after immobilization. Here, the priority is to drive the adaptation in the tissue and to recover motor control. If psychological factors are present, such as fear avoidance, they should also be addressed in the management.

SUMMARY

- This chapter discusses how to plan a ROM rehabilitation treatment using a functional approach and how to match the management to the patient's condition
- ROM challenges that contain effective ingredients from the recovery behaviour are likely to be more effective than approaches that have fewer of these components
- ROM challenges are likely to be more effective if they are task-specific, repetitive, active, provide overloading and use goal and whole movement

- Functional ROM challenges, including managed and assisted approaches, all contain the effective ingredients necessary for ROM adaptation
- Extra-functional ROM challenges, including all traditional passive and active stretching approaches, provide only a few or none of the effective ingredients
- Passive approaches provide no effective ingredients and may therefore, be least effective for ROM recovery
- ROM rehabilitation should strive to function at a level that matches the individual's movement capacity
- Regressing to a lower level, below the patient's current capacity, is likely to reduce effectiveness and may prolong recovery
- Joints should be challenged within their role in the overall movement of the limb and in the context of the movement repertoire of the individual
- Many daily activities can be exaggerated to challenge ROM losses at home. This should be the emphasis of the management
- Message to the patient - your everyday activities play a crucial role in your recovery

CHAPTER 13

Demonstration of Functional Approach in ROM Rehabilitation

This chapter explores the use of functional range of movement (ROM) rehabilitation within a clinical setting. The demonstration will focus on the ROM rehabilitation of the upper limb (shoulder and elbow) and trunk. The management approach described for these areas can be applied elsewhere in the body. The book is accompanied by a video demonstration of the ROM challengers, which can be viewed online at: www.therapeuticstretch.com.

GENERAL PRINCIPLES FOR FUNCTIONAL STRETCHING

There are several principles to consider during functional ROM challenges:

- Use movements that resemble normal daily activities
- Use external goals – provide instructions such as "Reach for my hand" or "Reach for the opposite wall". Avoid internal prompts such "Bend your elbow" or instructions that are directed to particular muscles. If internal instructions become necessary, incorporate them into the overall task, e.g. "While reaching for my hand try to straighten your elbow".
- Amplify the four movement parameters within the task, in particular the ones most affected
- Mix ranges and planes
- Mix end- with full-range challenges
- Mix dynamic and static tasks
- Mix all of the above – this will enhance generalization within the task

CONTENTS OF THE DEMONSTRATION

187

13.1. DEMONSTRATION OF PRINCIPLES

13.1.1 Amplifying the movement parameters during a dynamic task

Fig. 13.1A–D: Challenging the force parameter in the task, such as reaching and retrieving. Resistance can be provided by use of heavier objects or varying degrees of resistance from the therapist (See further in this chapter).

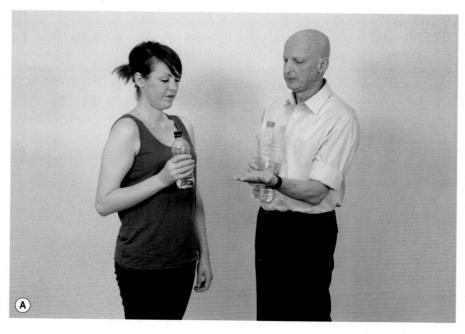

Ⓐ

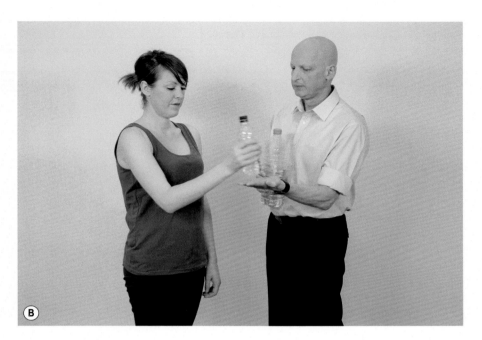

B

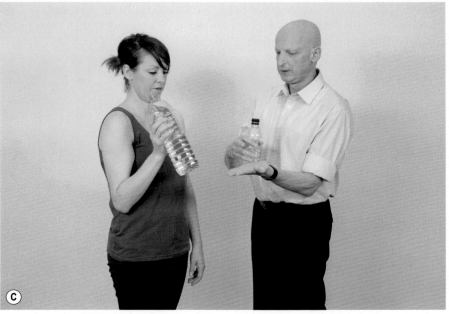

C

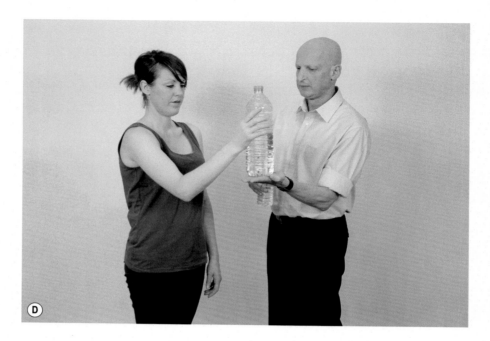

Fig. 13.2A–D: Challenging the range parameter with the reaching–retrieving task. Here, the range parameter is challenged within the same plane (range-on-range), flexion–extension.

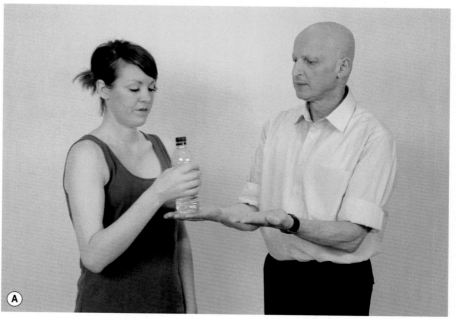

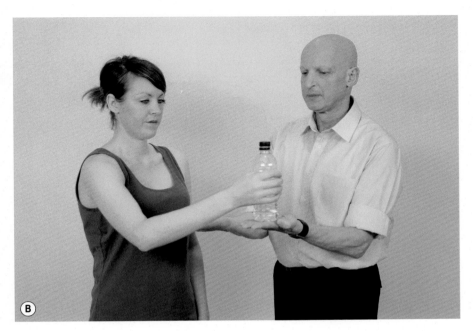

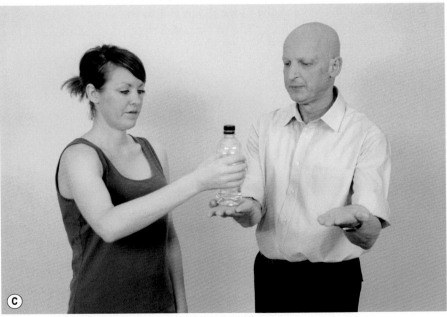

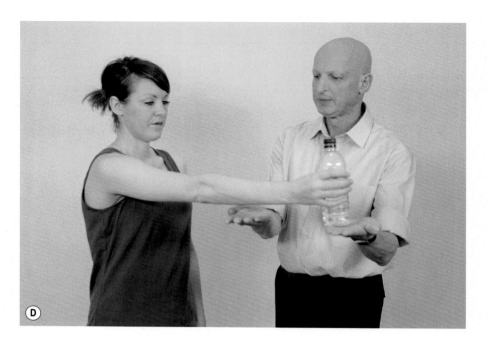

Fig. 13.3A,B: Challenging the range parameter of the same task but in a different plane, i.e. reaching and retrieving within abduction–adduction.

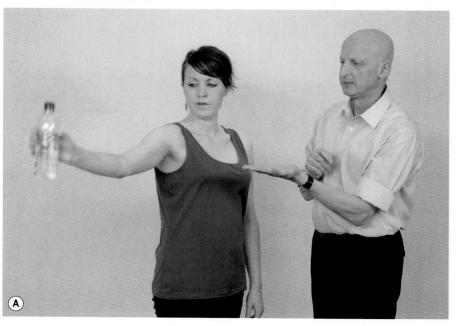

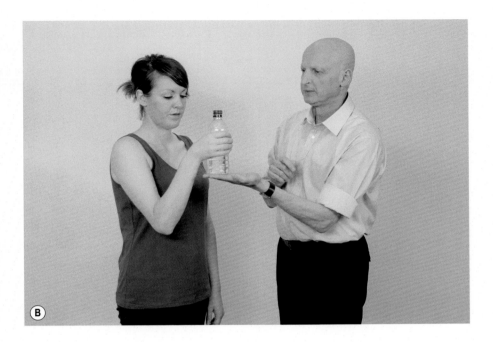

Notes on task parameters:

- For the velocity parameters any of the above movements can be performed at slower or greater speeds.
- The endurance parameter can be challenged by repetition of the same movement.
- Task parameters can be mixed. For example, the force can be combined with the velocity challenges, for instance by using the heavier bottle at progressively greater speeds.

13.1.2 Amplifying movement parameters during a static task

Fig. 13.4A–D. Many functional activities contain static tasks. This is reflected in challenges where the patient is instructed to hold the same position. In the following example the patient is instructed to hold the bottle and maintain it in the same position.

Fig. 13.4A,B: Challenging the force parameter during a static task.

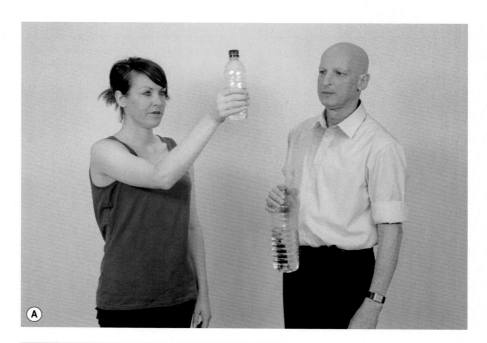

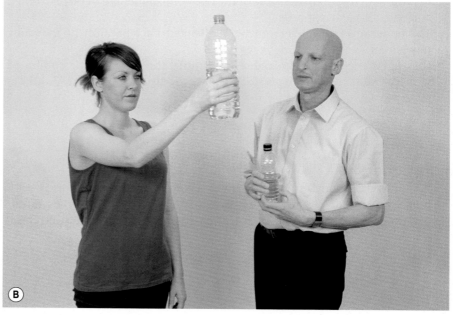

Fig. 13.4C: Here, the range parameter is challenged in different ranges, abduction and full flexion (in Fig. 13.4D).

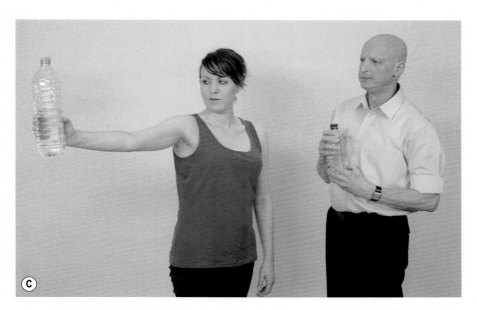

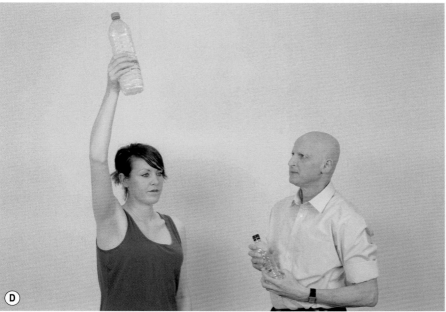

Notes about task parameters during static activities:

- Static endurance parameters can be challenged by maintaining the position for longer durations.
- Static velocity is how rapidly a person can generate a peak force while maintaining their position. This can be achieved by adding an external perturbation (by the therapist) while the patient maintains their position (see Fig. 13.16B). This challenge is demonstrated in the accompanying video.

13.1.3 Alternating between dynamic and static tasks

Fig. 13.5A,B: Alternating between a dynamic task (Fig. 13.5A) and a static task (Fig. 13.5B). In the dynamic task the patient is instructed to touch the therapist's hand. In the static task the patient is instructed to maintain the position and the therapist applies anterior–posterior perturbation in the same plane as the dynamic task. The alteration between dynamic and static task is often introduced at a progressively faster rate and can eventually be applied randomly.

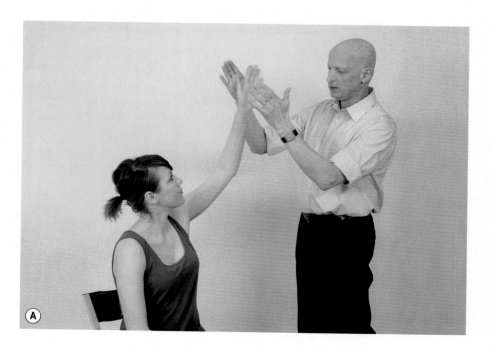

(A)

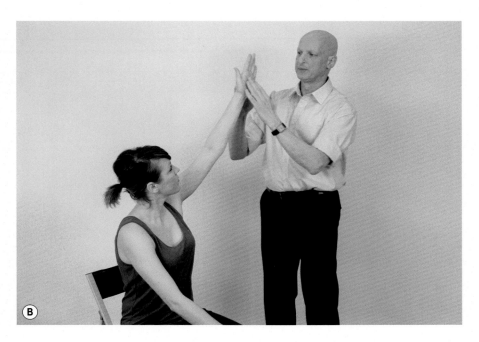

Fig. 13.6A,B: Another example of alternating between dynamic (Fig. 13.6A) and static (Fig. 13.6B) challenges. The instruction in the dynamic task is "Place the bottle on my hands", whereas in the static task the instruction is "Hold the bottle in the same position. Stop me from moving it".

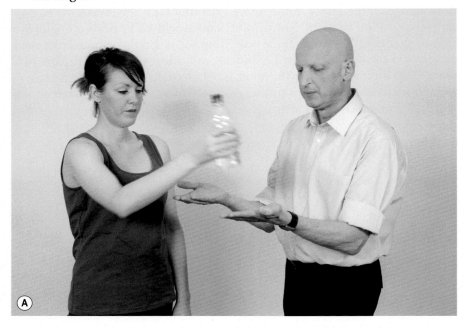

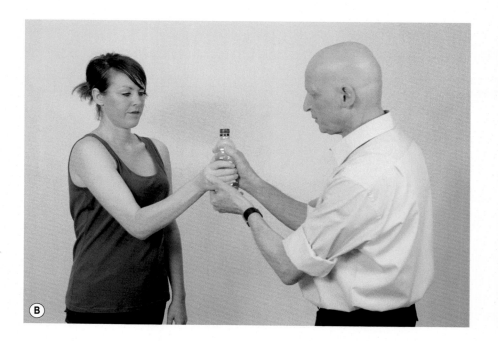

13.1.4 Context and localization of amplification

The contex principle suggests that tasks that typify arm movement can be used to challenge all the joints in the upper extremity (and the rest of the body). Some localization to specific areas/joints can be achived by positioning of the limb or changing the nature of the task. However, it should be noted that such localization of movement can be difficult to achieve clinically, in particular when ROM limitation in specific joints is compensated for by excessive movement in adjacent areas. This is further discussed in section 13.1.6 (overcoming compensatory movement patterns).

Fig. 13.7A,B: Localizing a dynamic challenge to the elbow. The therapist supports the patient's elbow and instructs them to gently tap the rolled up paper against the therapist's hand. This produces end-range flexion–extension cycles in the elbow with little dynamic activity from the shoulder (however, the shoulder is statically active).

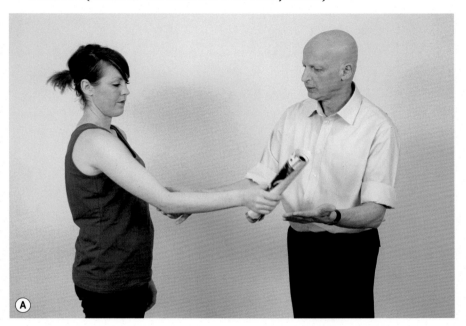

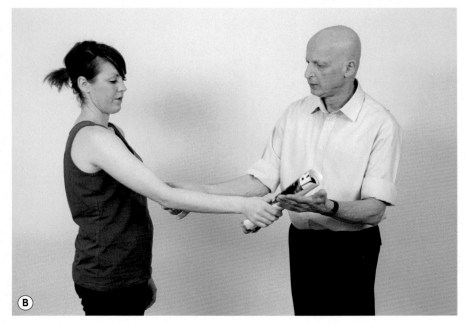

Fig. 13.8A,B: Localizing the dynamic challenge to the shoulder (flexion–extension cycles, but also in the elbow). The patient is instructed to alternately tap the rolled up paper between the therapist's hands.

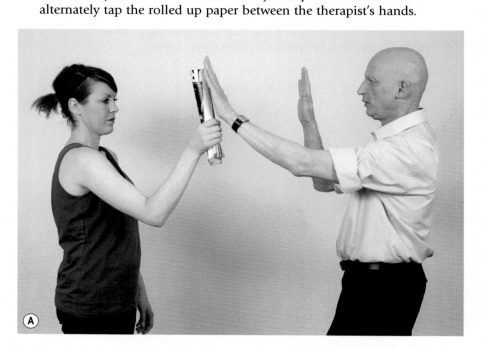

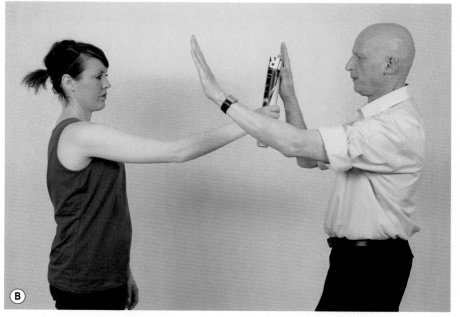

13.1.5 Mixing ranges and planes

Normal functional movement is highly variable and often involves multiple planes. Generalization of training may occur more readily when end-ranges are mixed with the whole-range challenges, as well as performing the same task in different planes (this is better demonstrated in the accompanying video).

Patients who are unable to perform a movement in a particular range can be still challenged in that range (primary challenge) but with movements in another plane (secondary challenge). This principle of primary and secondary challenges is demonstrated in this section.

> Fig. 13.9A–C: Imagine a clinical situation in which the patient is unable to elevate the arm in abduction above shoulder height. In this situation they are instructed to raise the arm to their end-range (primary challenge). While in that range they can be instructed to perform a movement challenge (secondary challenge). In this example, internal–external rotation (secondary challenge) is imposed on the abducted shoulder (primary challenge).

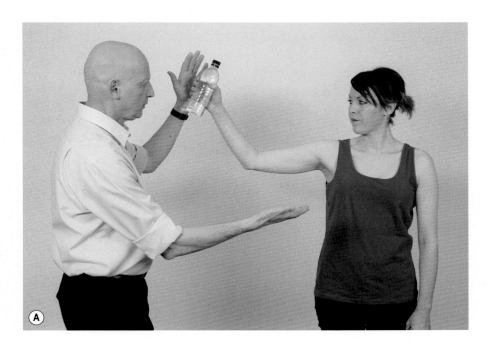

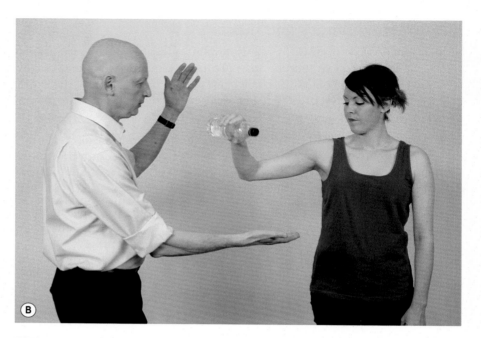

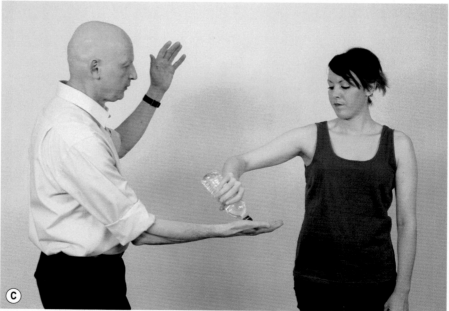

Fig. 13.10A–C: In this example, the primary challenge is external rotation with superimposed secondary abduction–adduction challenges.

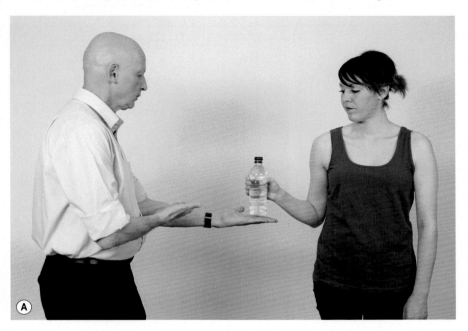

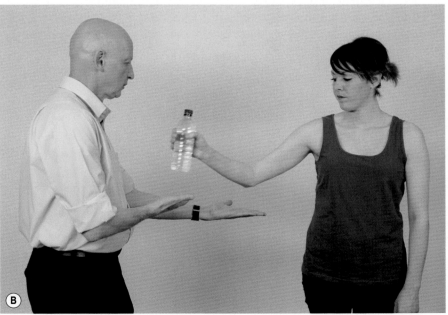

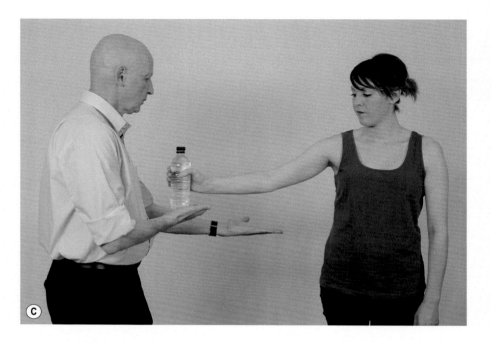

Fig. 13.11A–D: In this example, the primary challenge is internal rotation. The patient is instructed to imagine that they are "washing their back". This task produces secondary abduction–adduction cycles (superimposed on internal rotation).

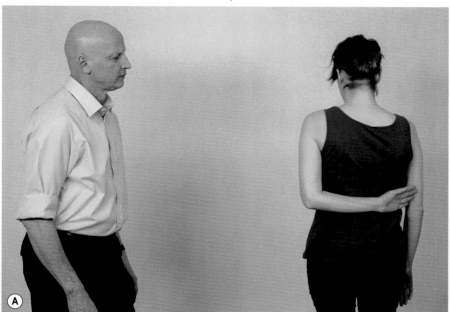

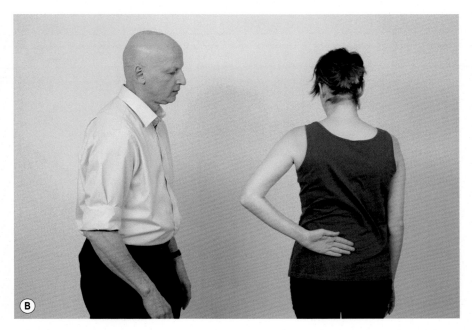

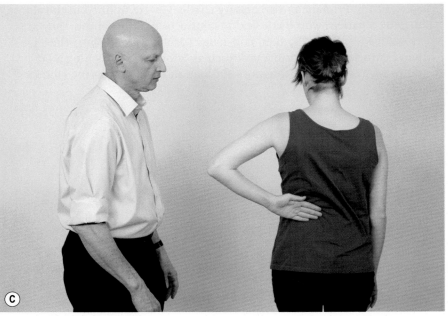

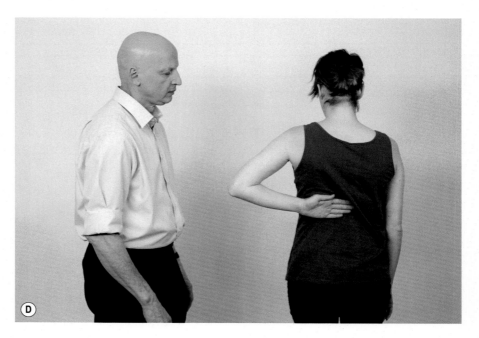

Fig. 3.12A,B: Primary and secondary challenges exemplified in the elbow. Imagine a patient who has a flexion contracture in the elbow. They are encouraged to extend to their end-range (primary challenge). They are then instructed to perform a task such as "closing and opening a lid", imposing a secondary pronation–supination challenge on the elbow.

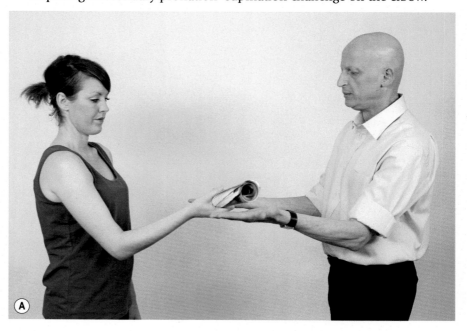

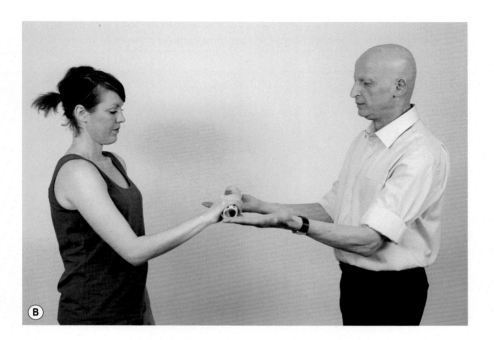

13.1.6 Overcoming compensatory movement patterns

One common problem with ROM loss is compensatory movement patterns elsewhere, which may reduce the efficacy of rehabilitation. Often, these compensatory patterns can be overcome by small modifications of the task, while keeping the focus of attention towards external goals.

Fig. 13.13A: A person with shoulder abduction ROM loss will often compensate by side-bending when reaching up (see angle between thorax and upper arm).

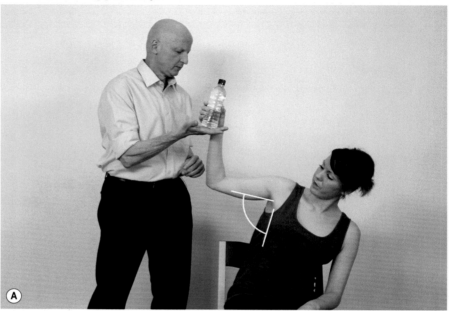

Fig. 13.13B: The compensatory side-bending can be overcome by placing the movement goal further to the side.

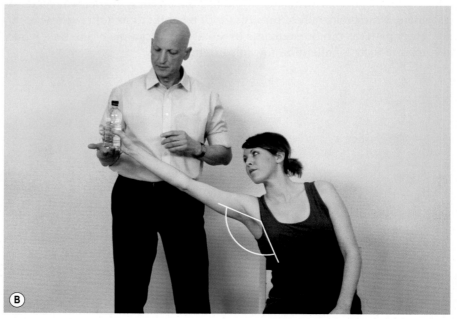

Fig. 13.14A: Shoulder flexion restrictions are often compensated for by the patient arching back.

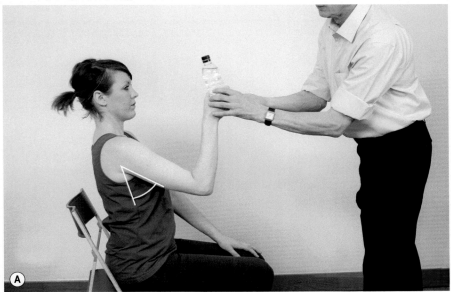

Fig. 13.14B: The extension compensation can be overcome by placing the movement goal further to the front.

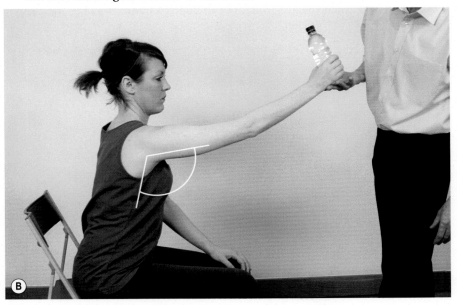

Fig. 13.15A: A movement such as reaching back is often compensated for by rotation of the whole body.

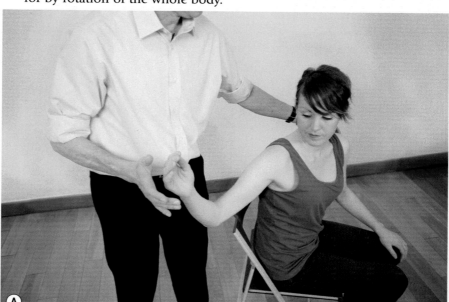

Fig. 13.15B: Trunk rotation can be overcome by instructing the patient to hold the back of the chair with the opposite arm. The patient is then instructed to reach over to touch the therapist's hand as in Fig. 13.15A

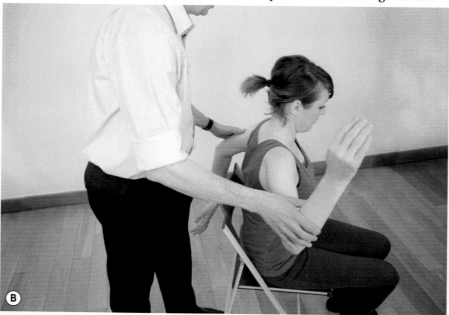

13.1.7 Therapist's stance and patient handling

Fig. 13.16A,B: Demonstrating the hand-hold in challenges in which the therapist is providing the resistance.

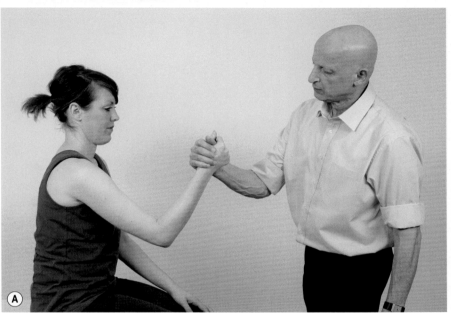

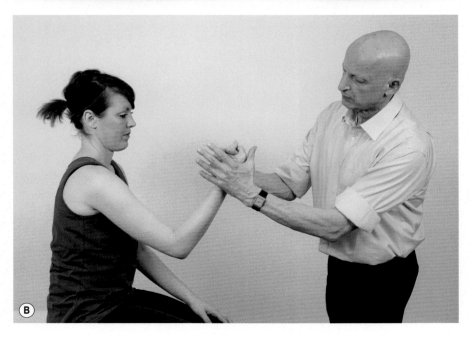

Fig. 13.17A,B: Keep the hand-hold close to your body, using your own body to provide the resistance force. Keep this close contact throughout the movement cycle.

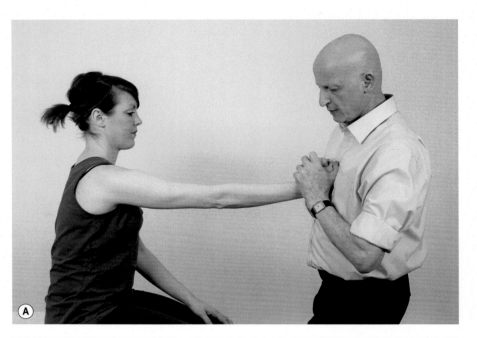

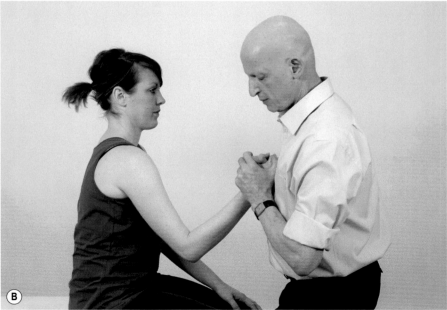

Fig. 13.18: Avoid hand-holds that are away from your body. Such hand-holds are more fatiguing for the therapist.

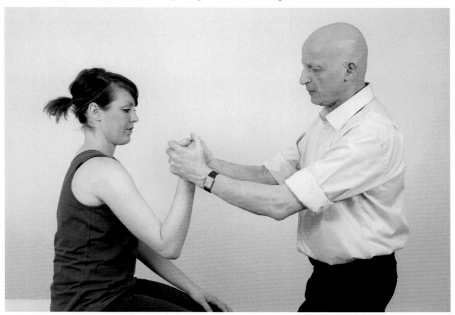

Fig. 13.19A,B: Throughout the movement cycle, shift your body weight between the legs. Avoid bending with your trunk or working with the top of your body.

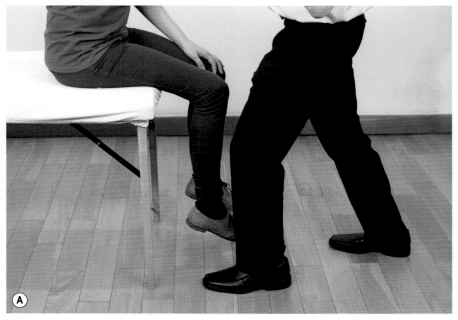

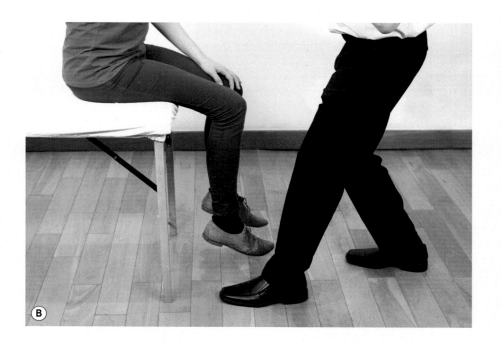

13.2. SHOULDER ROM CHALLENGES

13.2.1 ROM challenge during dynamic tasks

Fig. 13.20A–F: Range challenge/single plane/free movement/flexion–extension cycles. Demonstrating progressive increase in flexion range. Instructions to patient: "Reach and tap my hands".

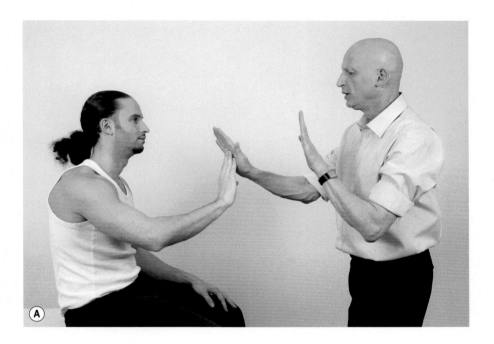

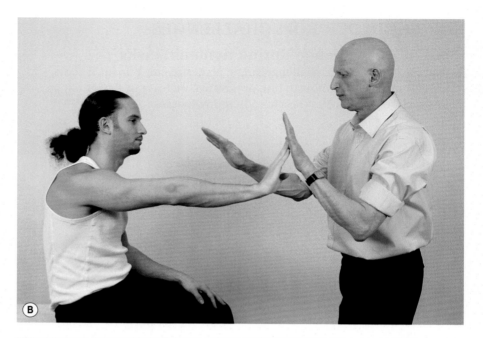

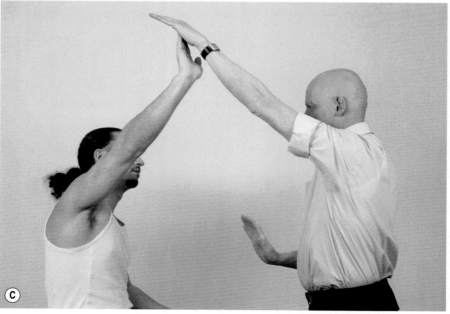

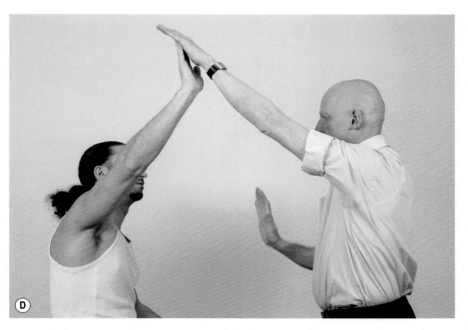

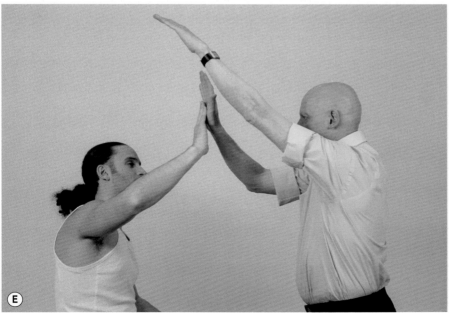

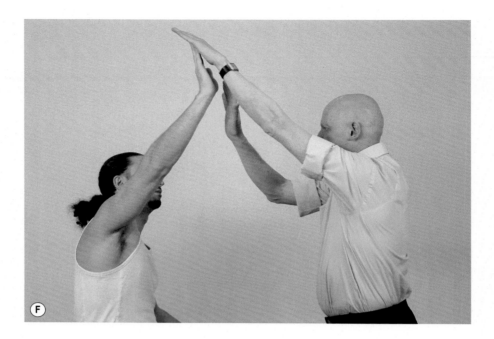

Fig. 13.21A,B: Range + force challenge/single plane/flexion–extension cycles. Instructions to patient: "Pull and push me".

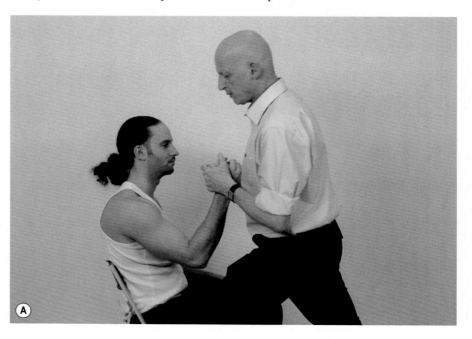

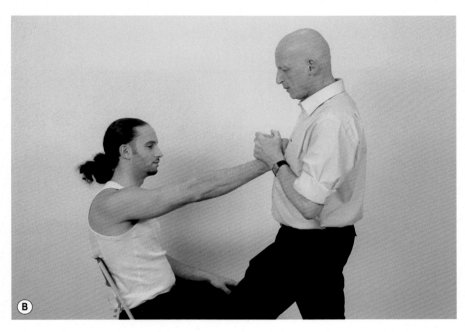

Fig. 13.22A–E: Range challenge/single plane/free movement/adduction–abduction cycles. Demonstrating progressive increase in abduction range. Instructions to patient: "Tap my hands".

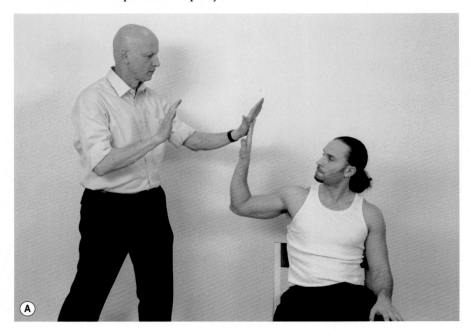

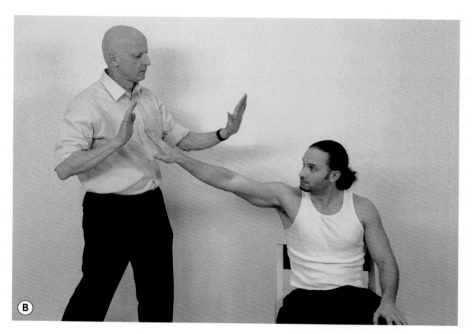

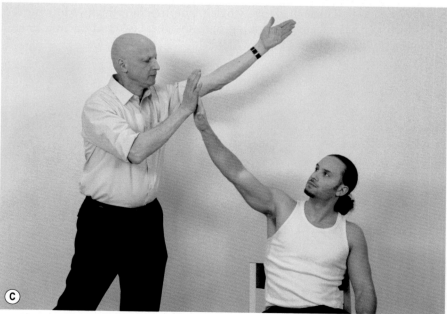

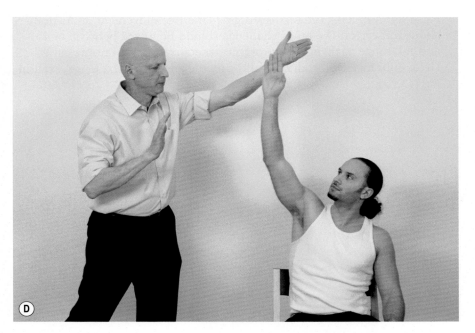

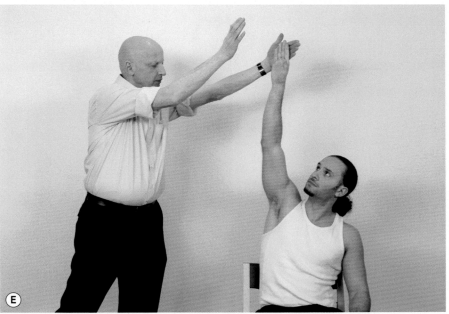

Fig. 13.23A,B: Range challenge/single plane/free movement/adduction–abduction cycles. The range challenge should be mixed between end- and full-range challenges to promote generalization of training gains. Here, full range is introduced following the end-range challenges seen in Fig. 13.22E.

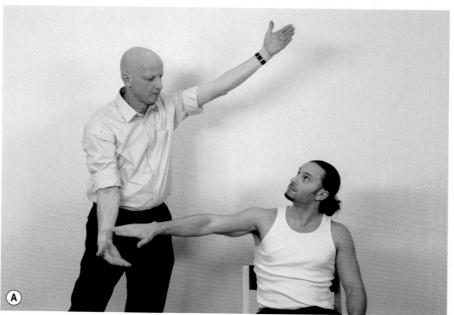

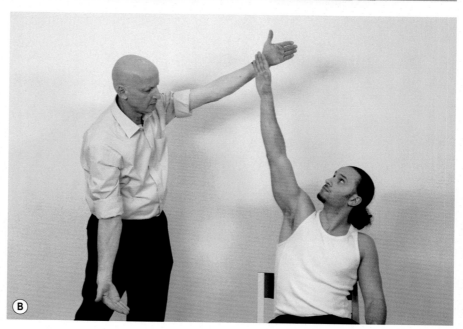

Fig. 13.24A,B: Range + force challenge/single plane/adduction–abduction cycles. Instructions to patient: "Pull and push me".

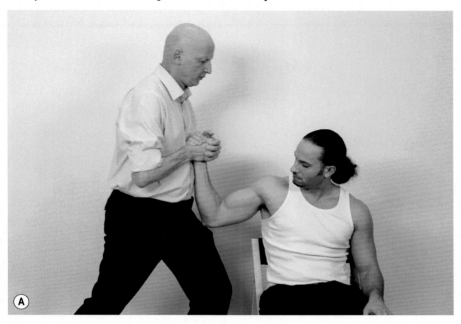

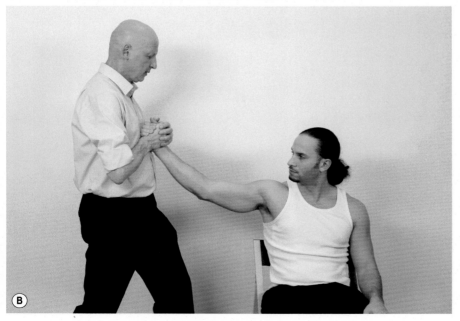

Note: hand-hold close to the body and the use of body weight to provide resistance.

Fig. 13.25A–D: Range challenge/single plane/free movement/internal–external rotation cycles. Demonstrating a progressive increase in shoulder rotation range. Instructions to patient: "Touch your tummy and then reach for my hand", or "Touch your tummy, and reach for the wall behind".

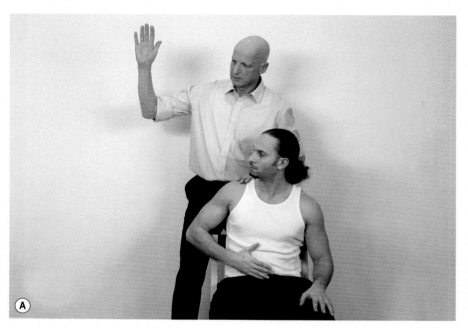

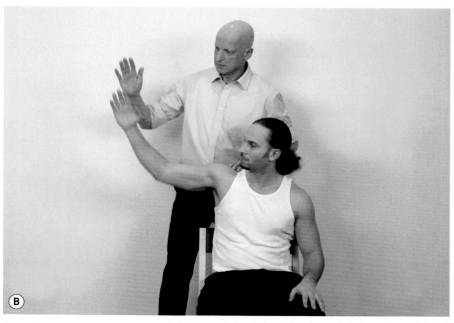

Fig. 13.25C: Note: patients tend to rotate with the trunk to compensate for loss of rotation range in the shoulder. This can be overcome by instructing the patient to hold the back of the chair with the opposite arm.

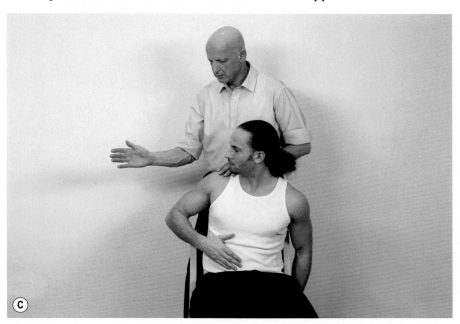

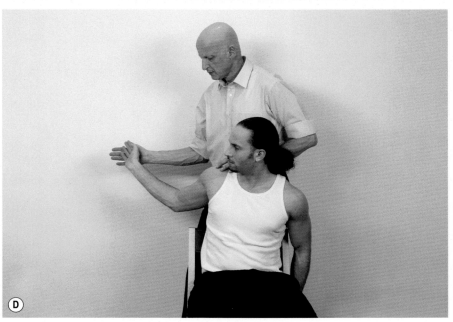

Fig. 13.26A,B: Range challenge/free movement/internal–external rotation cycles. Instructions to patient: "Touch your tummy, reach for my hand".

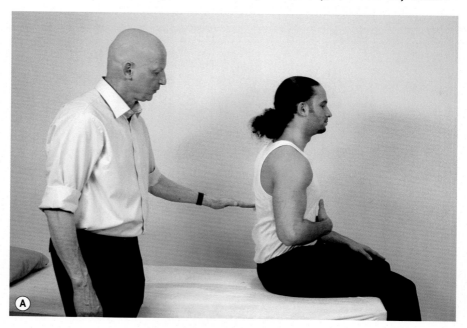

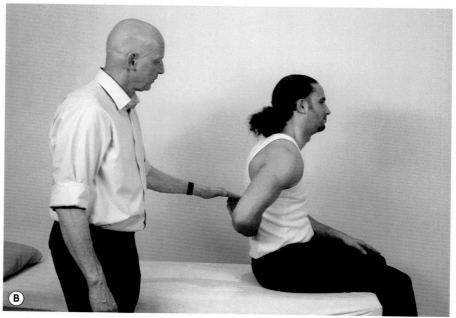

Fig. 13.27A–D: Range + force challenge/single plane/internal rotation cycles. Demonstrating the hand-hold: using the hand closer to the table, the therapist holds the patient's wrist. The elbow is supported with the other hand.

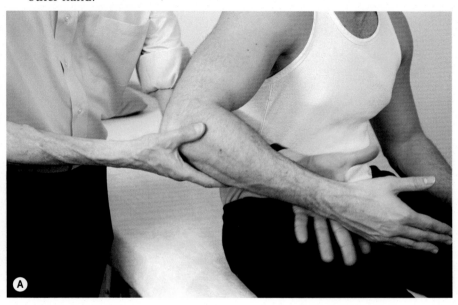

Fig. 13.27B: It is important that the therapist keeps their elbow tucked into the side of their body to provide resistance to the movement.

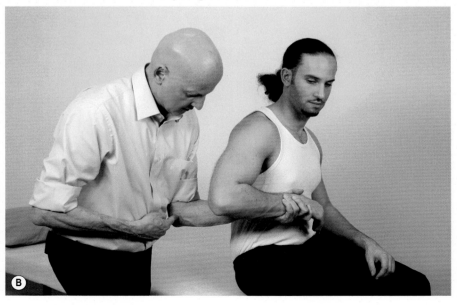

Fig. 13.27C: Throughout the movement, the therapist resists both internal and external rotation. Instructions to patient: "Touch your tummy, touch your back".

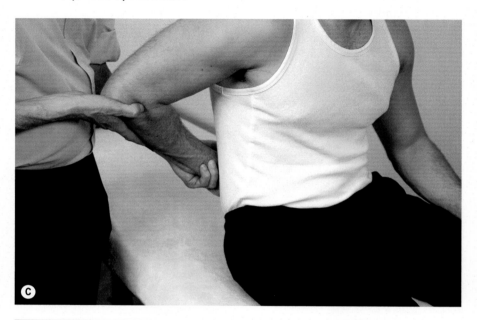

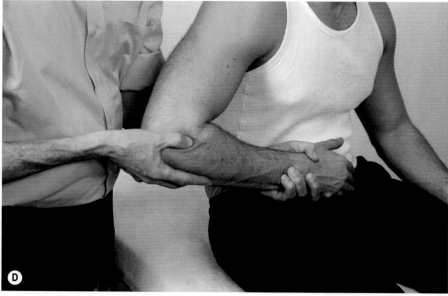

Fig. 13.28A–D: Range + force challenge/mixed planes/internal rotation to flexion cycles. Therapist provides resistance through the cycle. Instructions to patient: "Touch your back, reach for my hand".

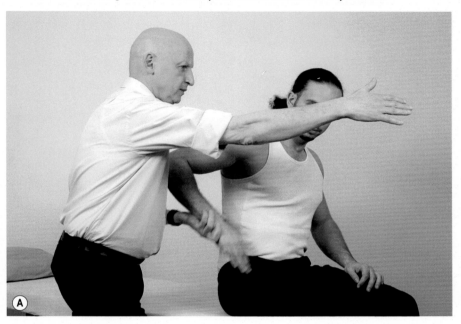

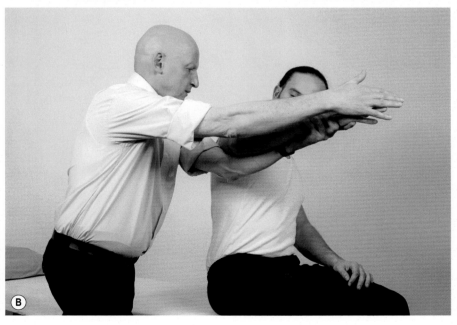

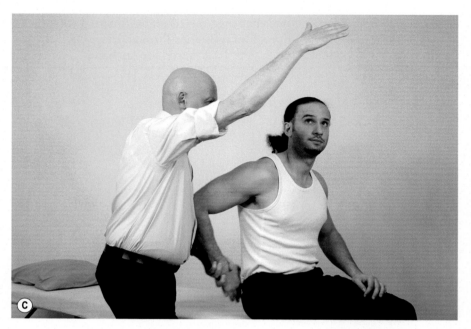

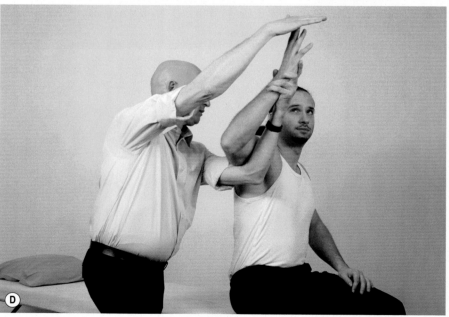

Fig. 13.29A,B: Range + force challenge/mixed planes/internal rotation to abduction cycles. Therapist provides resistance throughout the cycle. Instructions to patient: "Touch your back, reach for my hand".

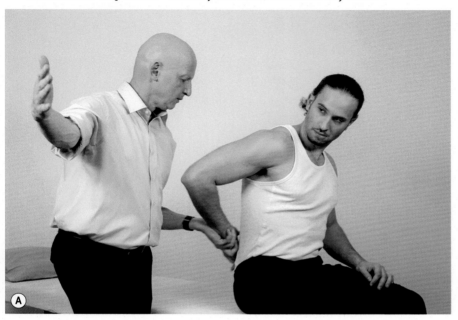

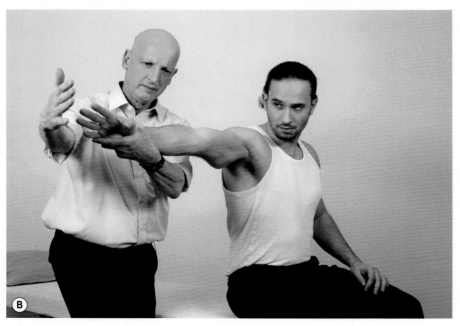

Fig. 13.30A,B: Range + force challenge/mixed planes/internal–external rotation cycles. Therapist provides resistance throughout the cycle. Instructions to patient: "Touch your back, touch the top of your head".

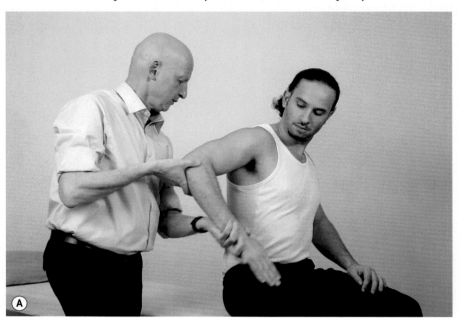

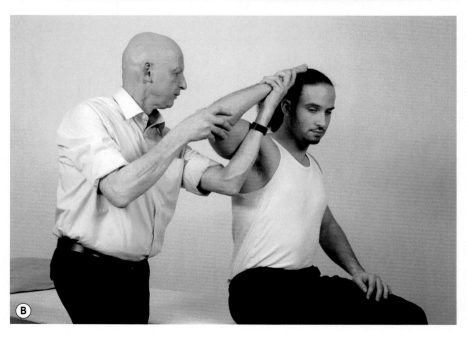

Fig. 13.31A: Seated position shoulder challenges. Demonstration of therapist stance and patient handling. The therapist rests the length of their forearm along the upper border of the patient's scapula, to reduce excessive scapular compensation/elevation during overhead arm movements. The therapist's hip should be in contact with the lateral border of the scapula to further reduce scapular winging.

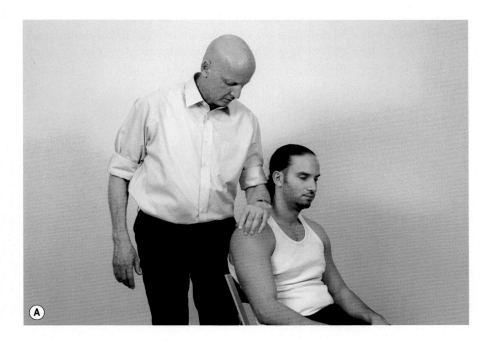

Fig. 13.31B: Demonstration of hand-hold. Instructions to patient: "Reach for the ceiling" (Fig. 13.31B), "Reach for your head" (Fig. 13.31C), "Reach for the wall beside you" (Fig. 13.31D) and "Reach to the wall in front" (Fig. 13.31E). Therapist provides resistance throughout the movements. Once in full flexion (primary challenge), the patient can be instructed to "Draw circles on the ceiling" (circumduction movement), "Imagine you are waving a flag" (adduction–abduction movements), "Imagine you are painting the ceiling" (flexion–extension movement), or "Draw numbers from 0 to 10 on the ceiling" (combination of movements). Variation: draw larger numbers, more vigorous large-amplitude waving, etc. Mix the sequence of all these movements.

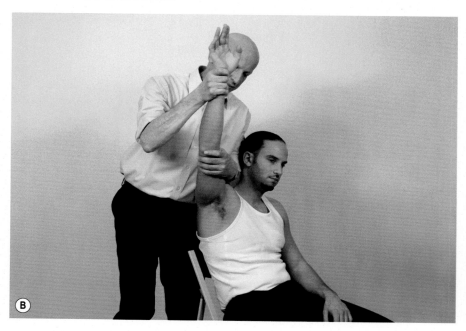

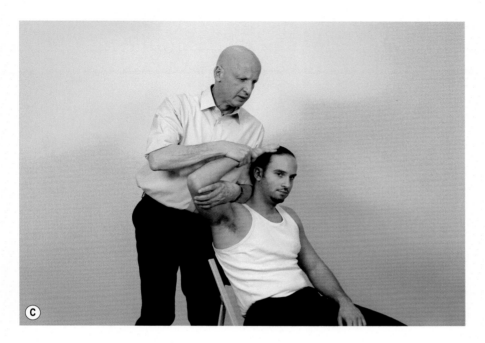

Fig. 13.31D: Once in abduction the patient can be instructed to "Draw circles on the wall to the side", "Imagine you are painting the wall" or "Draw numbers from 0 to 10 on the wall to the side". In essence, the instruction should be associated with daily tasks that challenge the particular movement patterns.

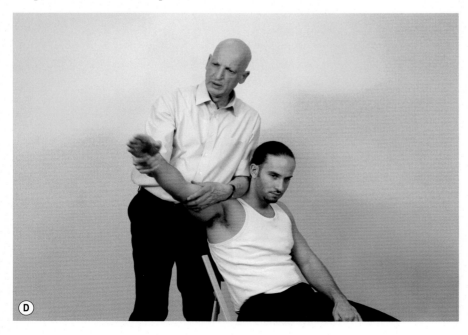

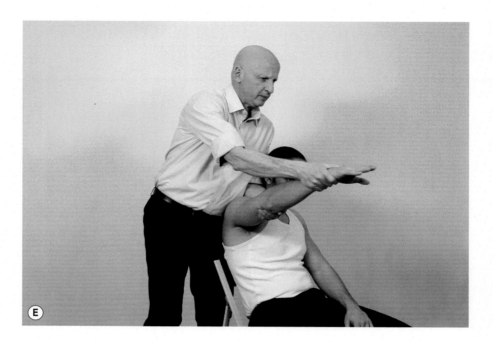

Fig. 13.32: Range + force/primary challenge internal rotation/secondary challenge adduction–abduction. Instructions to patient: "Wash your back" or "Pull and push me".

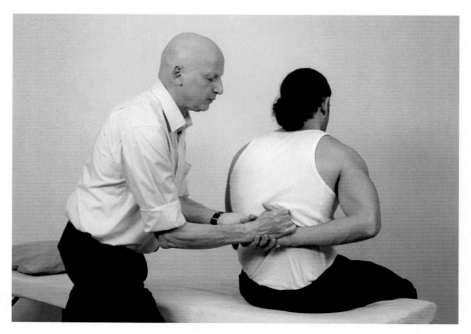

13.2.2 ROM challenges during static tasks

Fig. 13.33A,B: Range + force/static/flexion–extension cycles. Patient maintains position while the therapist introduces perturbations in the lateral plane. Instructions to patient: "Hold your arm in this position. Stop me from moving you".

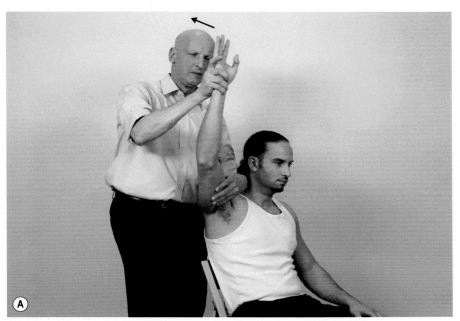

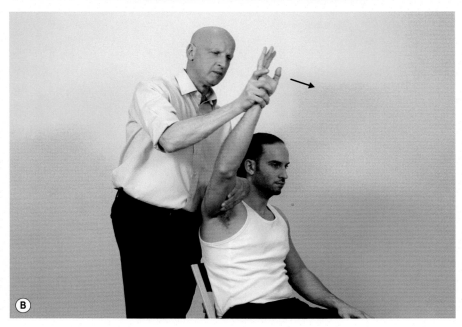

Fig. 13.34A,B: Range + force/static/abduction–adduction cycles. Patient maintains position while the therapist introduces perturbations in the lateral plane. Instructions to patient: "Hold your arm in this position. Stop me from moving you."

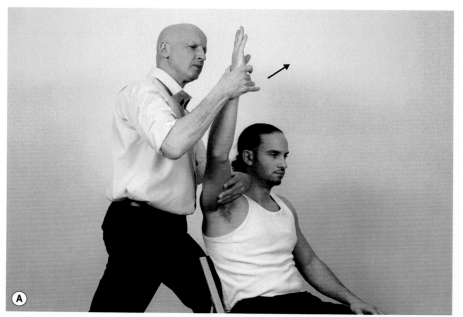

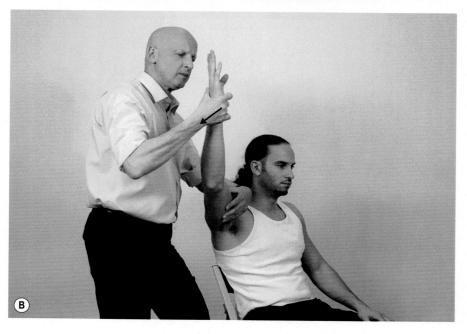

13.2.3 Guided challenge within a functional task

The guided challenges are the most important group in ROM rehabilitation as they closely resemble normal daily challenges of reaching and retrieving. A close resemblance between the clinical challenges and the affected functional tasks can help the patient conceptualize and apply the ROM rehabilitation principles in their home and work environment.

Fig. 13.35A–D: Range + (low) force/free movement/flexion–extension cycles. Demonstrating progressive increase in flexion range. Instructions to patient: "Place the bottle on my hands" or "Move the bottle from one shelf to another".

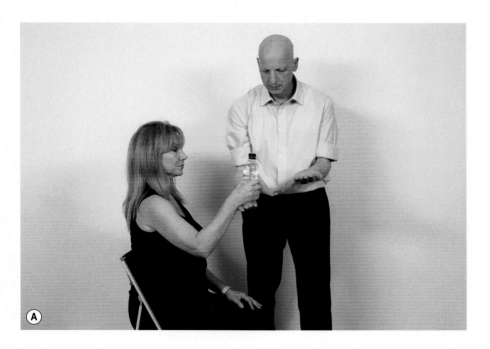

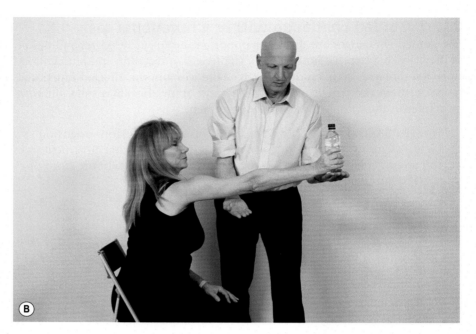

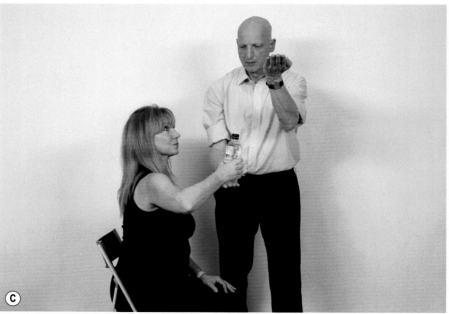

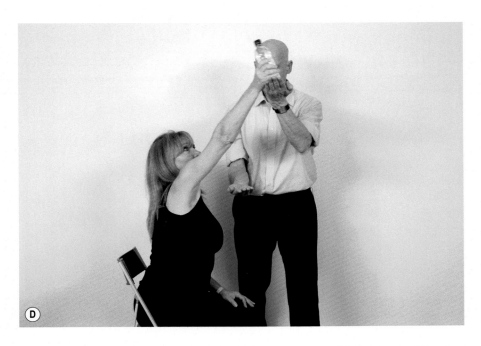

Fig. 13.36A–C: Range + (low) force/free movement/abduction–adduction cycles. Demonstrating progressive increase in abduction range. Instructions to patient: "Place the bottle on my hands" or "Move the bottle from one shelf to another".

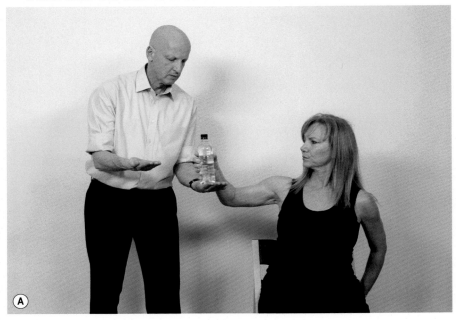

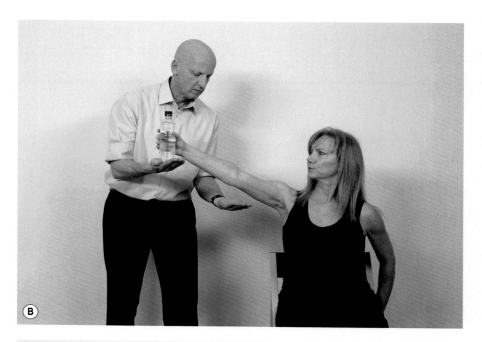

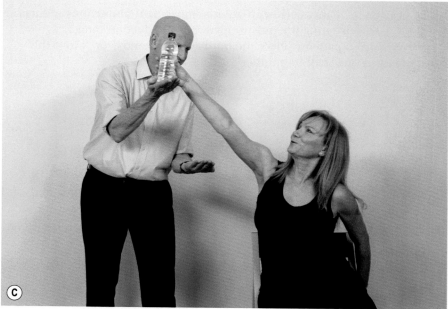

Fig. 13.37A,B : Range/primary challenge abduction/secondary challenge internal–external rotation. Instructions to patient: "Put the bottle on the shelf and then pour it onto the other hand".

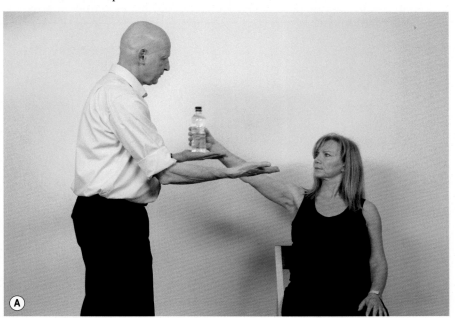

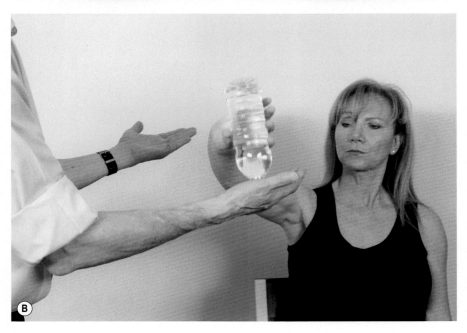

Fig. 13.38A–D: Range + force/flexion–extension cycles. The therapist instructs the patient to "Put the bottle on the hand/shelf" while providing resistance throughout the upward and downward movement. Variations: this challenge can also be performed in abduction–adduction ranges, rotation, etc.

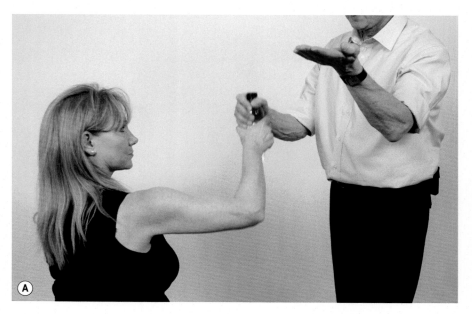

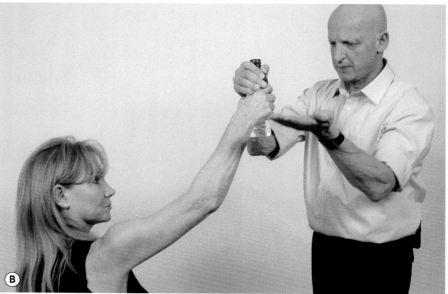

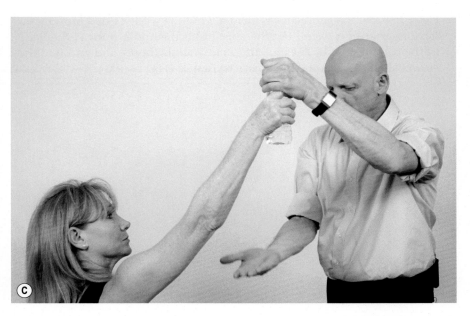

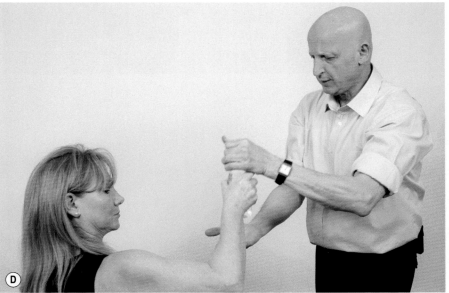

Fig. 13.39A,B: Range/free movement alternating with resisted movement/ flexion–extension cycles. The therapist holds the bottle at the end-range of the patient's reach. The patient has to grab the bottle and pull it to the "lower shelf" against the therapist's resistance (Fig. 13.39B).

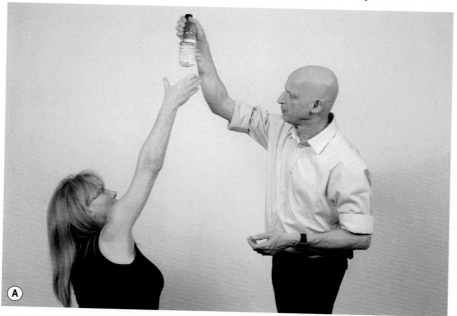

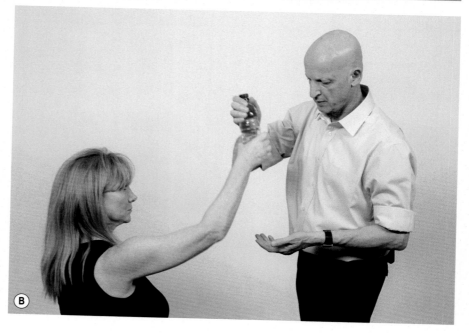

Fig. 13.40A,B: Range/free movement alternating with resisted movement/ abduction–adduction cycles. The therapist holds the bottle at the end-range of the patient's reach. The patient has to grab the bottle and pull it down to the "lower shelf" against the therapist's resistance (Fig. 13.40B).

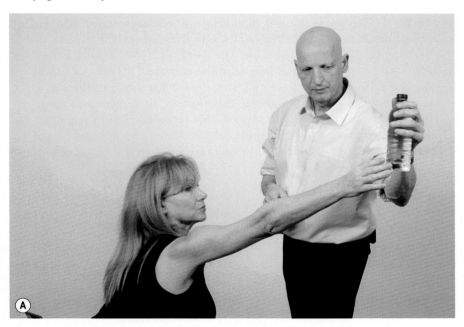

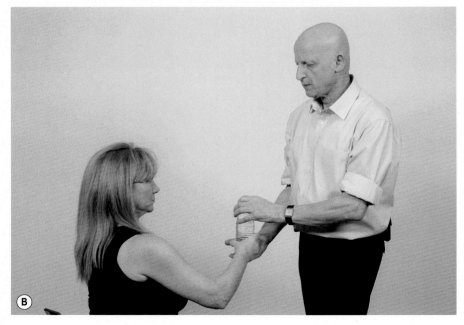

13.2.4 Assisted supine ROM challenges

Assisted supine techniques can be useful to localize the tissue loading to the glenohumeral joint. This is particularly useful in shoulder conditions in which there are excessive compensatory scapular movements owing to glenohumeral contractures (e.g. frozen shoulder).

Fig. 13.41: Patient positioning, handling and operator stance. The patient is positioned on the table diagonally with their affected shoulder overhanging the edge of the table. The therapist makes contact with their hip and the patient's lateral border of the scapula. This serves to limit scapular protraction–abduction. Using the fist the therapist then depresses the scapula from above. The therapist then leans and rests their fist firmly into the table surface. This serves to prevent scapular elevation. At this point the scapula is locked into position and movement of the shoulder will largely take place in the glenohumeral joint.

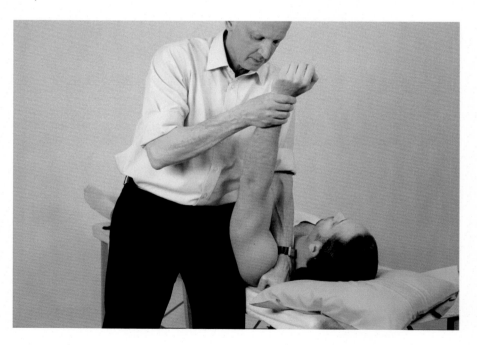

Fig. 13.42: Range/free movement/primary challenge flexion. From the locked position described in Fig 13.41, the patient is instructed to reach to the wall behind and given instructions such as "Draw circles on the wall behind" or "Draw numbers from 1 to 10".

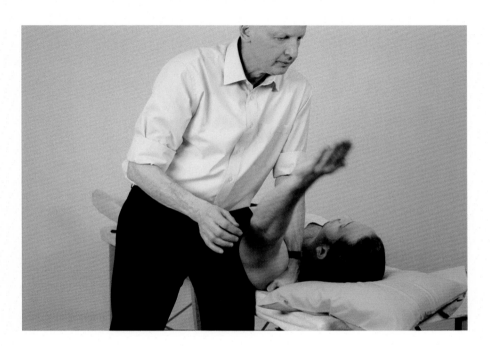

Fig. 13.43: Range/free movement/primary challenge abduction. From the locked position described in Fig 13.41, the patient is instructed to reach to the wall to the side. In this position they are given instructions such as "Draw circles on the wall behind" or "Draw numbers from 1 to 10".

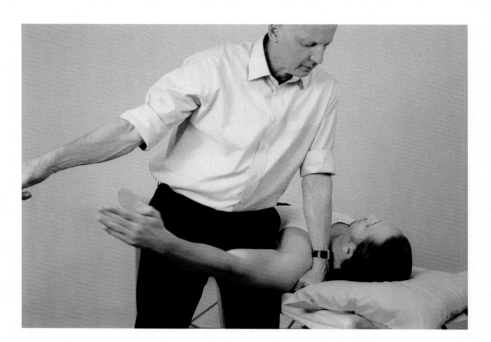

Fig. 13.44: Range + force/primary challenge flexion. The scapula is locked in position as in Fig 13.41. The therapist holds and resists the patient's arm movements. In this position, the patient is instructed to reach to the wall behind and given instructions such as "Draw circles on the wall behind", "Draw numbers from 1 to 10", "Imagine you are waving a flag", etc.

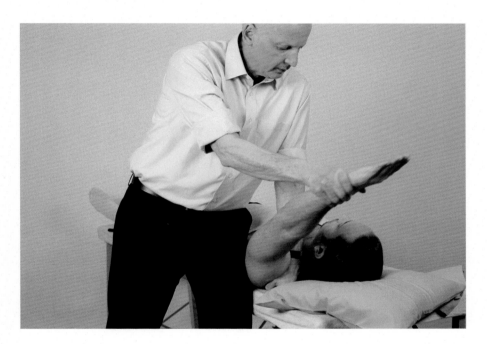

Fig. 13.45: Range + force/primary challenge abduction. Scapular locking: as in Fig. 13.41. Resistance and instructions to patient: as in Fig. 13.44.

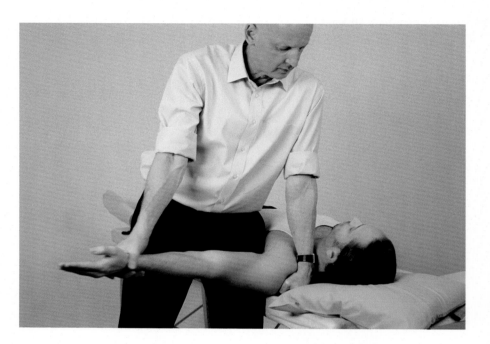

Fig. 13.46: Range + force/external rotation to abduction and flexion. The patient is instructed to touch the top of their head (external rotation) while the therapist provides resistance throughout the range. From this position, the patient is instructed to touch the wall behind (external rotation to flexion) or the wall to the side (external rotation to abduction). This challenge can be mixed with the static challenges or with challenges such as drawing numbers on the wall to the side or behind the patient.

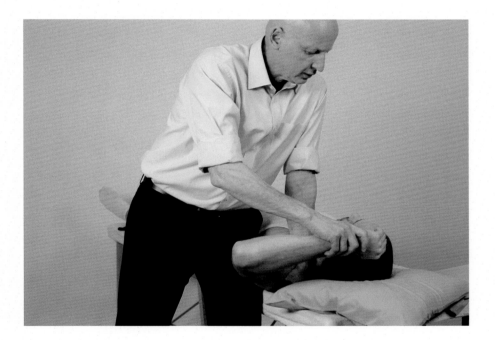

Fig. 13.47A,B: When glenohumeral contractures are present the patient may experience difficulties in touching their head while maintaining external rotation. The therapist can reinforce/assist the external rotation by holding the elbow down while the patient attempts the movement.

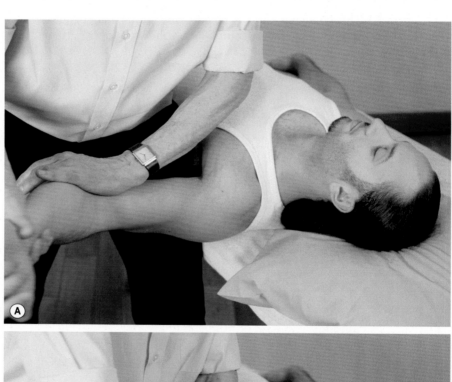

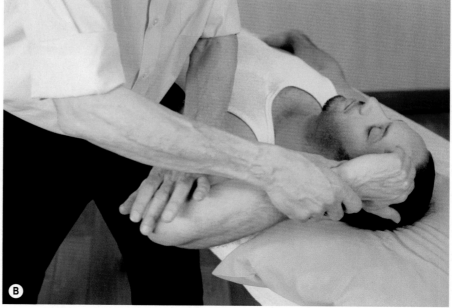

Fig. 13.48A,B: Range + force/flexion–extension cycles. In this position, the shoulder is taken into full possible flexion and the patient is instructed to perform small amplitude flexion–extension cycles against the therapist's resistance. Note the therapist's hand-hold and position, using their body weight to provide the resistance. Instructions to patient: "Push me away and then pull me towards you", "Repeat this movement".

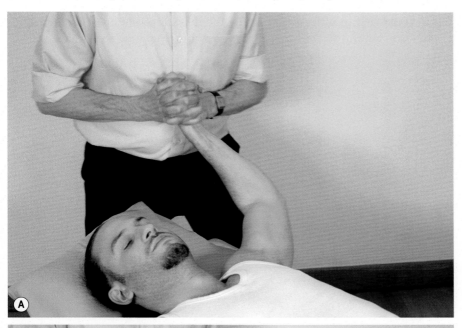

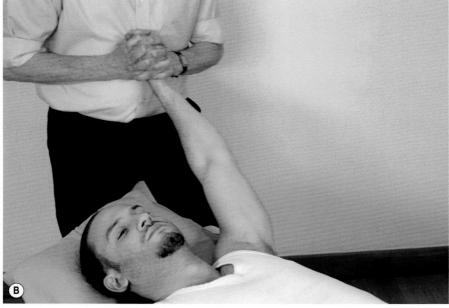

Fig. 13.49A,B: Range + force/abduction–adduction cycles. In this position, the shoulder is taken into full possible abduction and the patient is instructed to perform small-amplitude abduction–adduction cycles against the therapist's resistance. Note the therapist's hand-hold and position, using their body weight to provide the resistance. Instructions to patient: "Push me away and then pull me towards you", "Repeat this movement". Variation: this small end-range movement can be challenged in different ranges by the therapist walking in an arc from standing behind to standing to the side of the patient (see video).

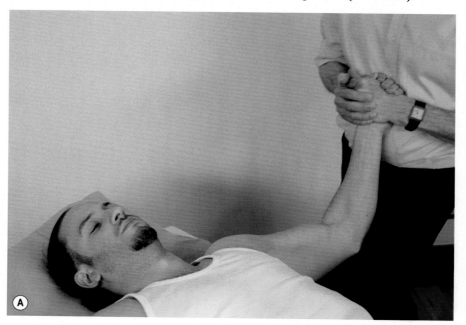

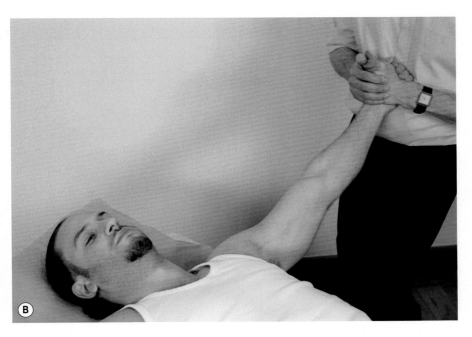

Fig. 13.50A,B: Range + force/primary challenge: abduction/secondary challenge: flexion–extension cycles. The shoulder is abducted to the possible end-range. In this position, the patient is instructed to push up towards the ceiling (flexion) and pull down towards the floor (extension). The therapist provides resistance throughout the movement. As the condition improves, the shoulder can be taken further into abduction.

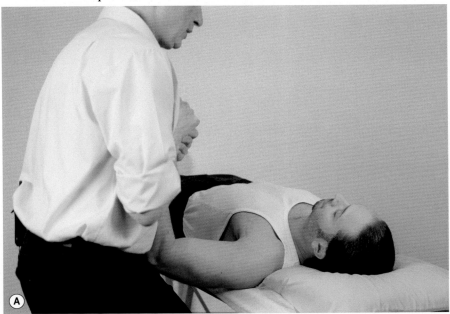

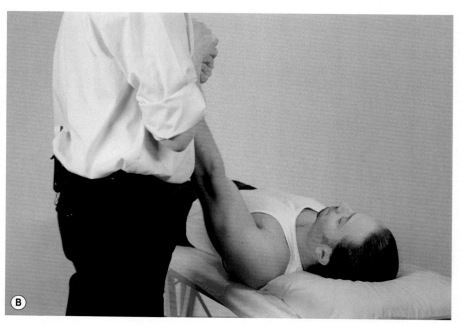

Note the therapist's hand-hold and position, and use of body weight to provide resistance.

13.3. ELBOW ROM CHALLENGES

Fig. 13.51A,B: Range/free movement/primary challenge: elbow extension/ secondary challenge: pronation–supination. The elbow is extended to the full possible end-range. In this position, the patient is instructed to "Open and close the lid" from one hand to the other.

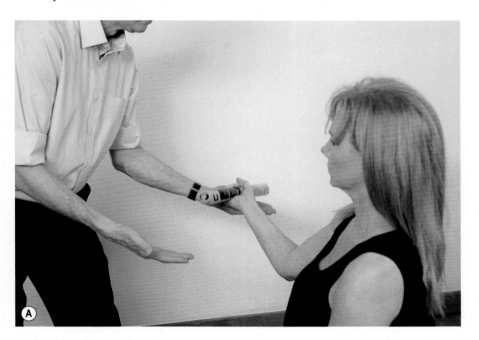

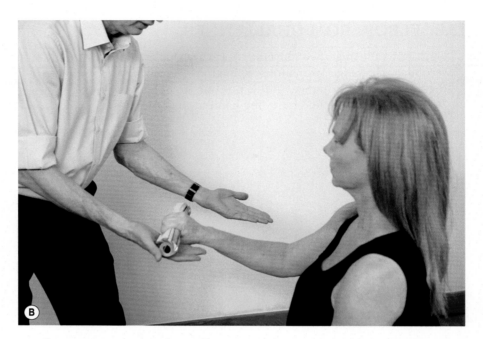

Fig. 13.52: Range + velocity/free movement/primary challenge: elbow extension/secondary challenge: pronation. The elbow is extended to the full possible end-range. Holding a paper roll by the end, the patient is instructed to tap the therapist rapidly and repeatedly. In conditions in which pronation is limited, the elbow may need to be supported to reduce compensatory internal rotation of the shoulder.

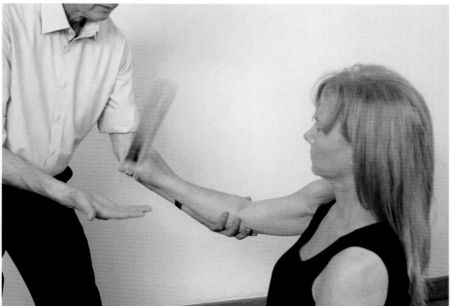

Fig. 13.53: Range + velocity/free movement/primary challenge: elbow extension/secondary challenge: supination. The elbow is extended to the full possible end-range. Holding a paper roll, the patient is instructed to tap the therapist rapidly and repeatedly. In conditions in which supination is limited the elbow may need to be supported to reduce compensatory movement of the shoulder.

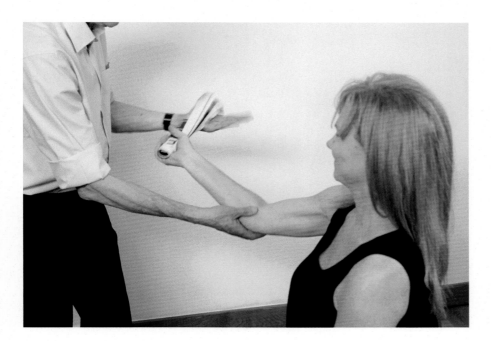

Fig. 13.54A,B: Range + force/primary challenge: elbow extension/ secondary challenge: elbow pronation–supination. The elbow is extended to the full possible end-range. Holding a paper roll by the middle, the patient is instructed to "Open and close the lid" repeatedly. The therapist provides resistance throughout the movement.

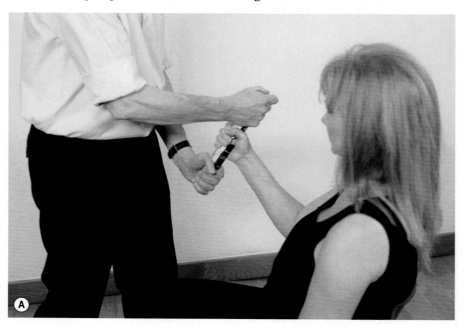

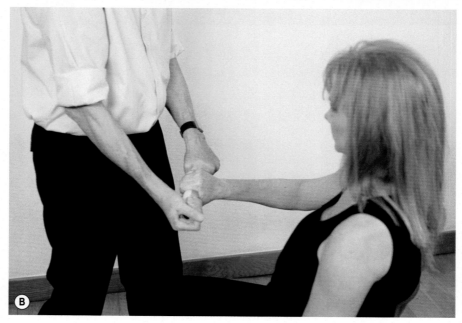

Fig. 13.55: Range + force/primary challenge: supination/secondary challenge: elbow flexion–extension cycles. Instruction to patient: "In this position pull me towards you and then push me away from you".

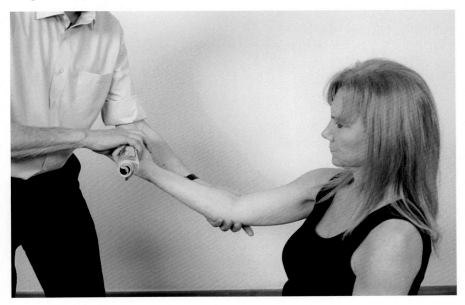

Fig. 13.56: Range/free movement/primary challenge: supination/secondary challenge: elbow flexion–extension cycles. Instruction to patient: "Maintain the hand position, tap my top and bottom hand".

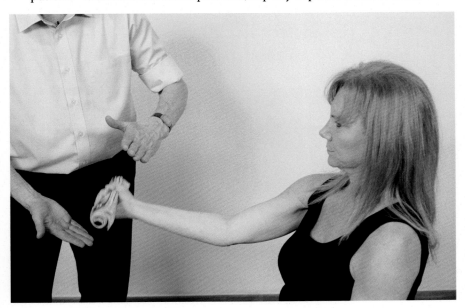

Fig. 13.57: Range/free movement/primary challenge: pronation/ secondary challenge: elbow flexion–extension cycles. Instruction to patient: "Tap my hand".

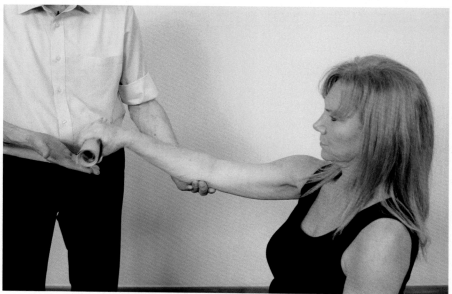

Fig. 13.58A,B: Range + velocity/free movement/flexion–extension cycles at end-range. Instructions to patient: "Tap my hand with the paper roll as fast as you can".

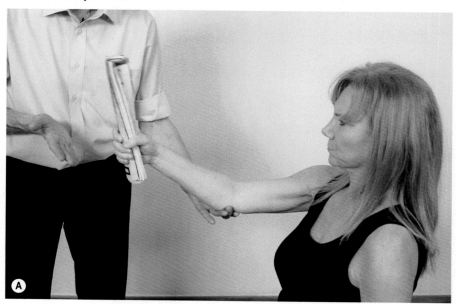

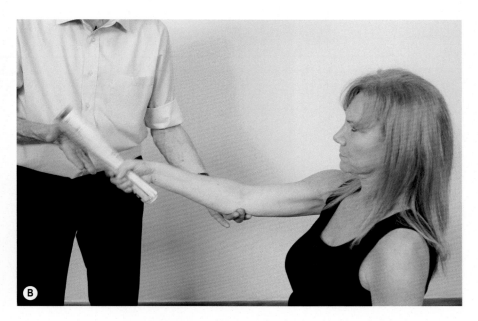

Fig. 13.59A,B: Range + force/primary challenge: flexion–extension (or supination)/secondary challenge: supination (or flexion–extension). Instructions to patient: "Push and pull me". Variation: to add the force parameter, use another target and instruct the patient to hit it as hard as they can.

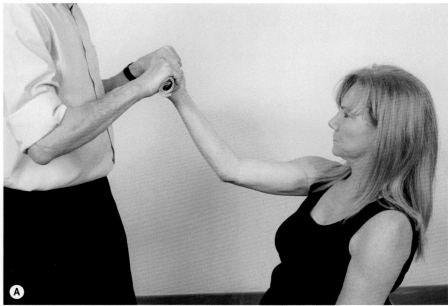

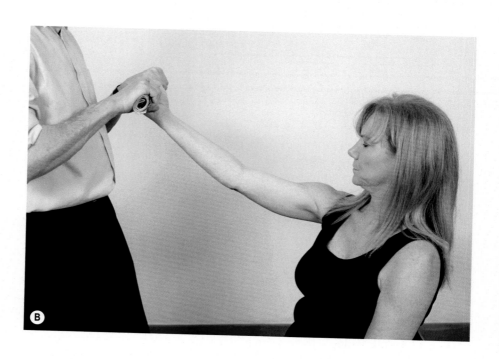

Fig. 13.60A,B: Range + force/primary challenge: flexion–extension (or pronation)/secondary challenge: pronation (or flexion–extension). Instructions to patient: "Push and pull me".

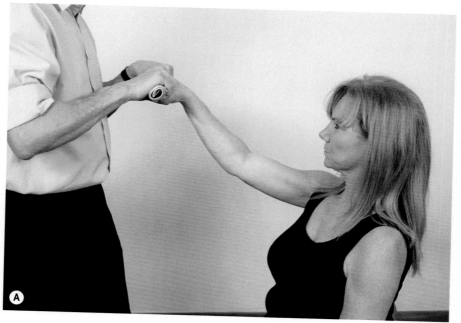

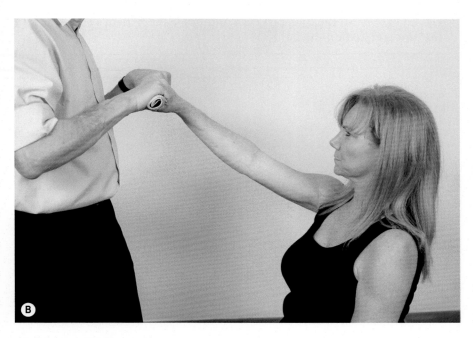

13.3.1 Assisted supine

Assisted supine elbow challenges are useful for localizing the force to that joint and to reduce excessive compensatory shoulder movements.

> Fig. 13.61A: Close-up of the practitioner's handling position and stance. The therapist fixes the patient's shoulder with their forearm. This will check compensatory movement of the shoulder.

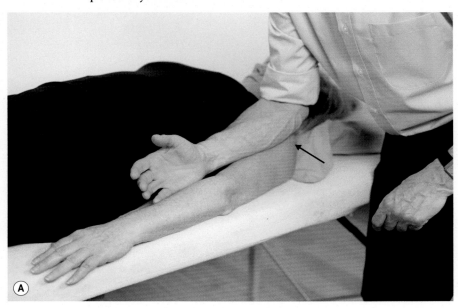

Fig. 13.61B: Next, the therapist cups and holds the patient's elbow and the arm is rested on the table.

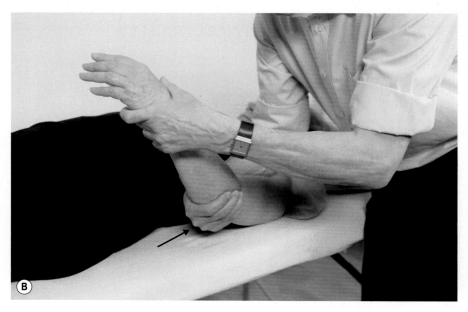

Fig. 13.62: Range + force/flexion–extension cycles. In this position the patient is instructed: "Reach for the top of the table and then to the shoulder; keep repeating that movement".

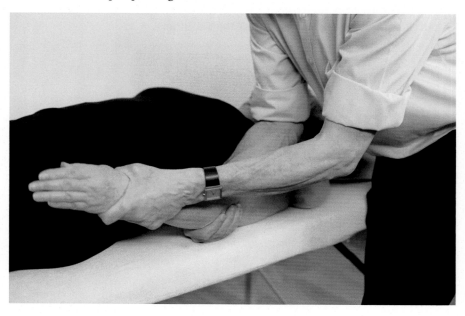

Fig. 13.63A,B: Range + force/primary challenge: flexion–extension cycles/ secondary challenge: pronation–supination. The elbow is extended to the possible end-range. Instructions to patient: "Touch your tummy. Touch the table with the back of your hand" (Fig. 13.62B).

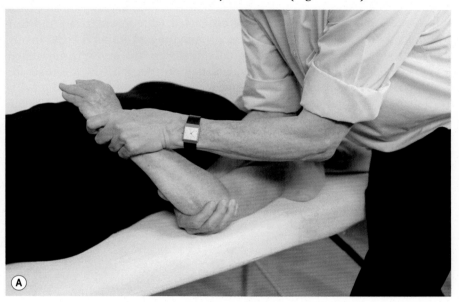

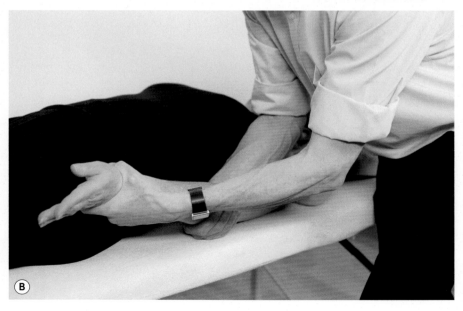

13.4. TRUNK ROM CHALLENGES

13.4.1 Standing challenges

The trunk challenges serve two purposes: to challenge end-range and to promote ROM desensitization. It is well established that, in many chronic back pain conditions, ROM losses may be associated with sensitization and fear avoidance rather than true shortening or stiffening of joints/tissues. In my clinical experience it is very rare to see individual who have severe tissue related spinal ROM losses. Often the challenges demonstrated below are used for trunk ROM desensitization. These challenges are preformed within the pain-free ranges. During successive cycles, the therapist (surreptitiously) moves the target further away to increase the range. Often, there is an increase in the pain-free end-range after a few repetitions of the same movement. This form of challenge can also be used to reassure the patient that the movement is safe (Ch. 11).

Fig. 13.64A,B: Range/free movement/rotation. Instructions to patient: "Keep the hands together, keep the arm straight. Touch my hands".

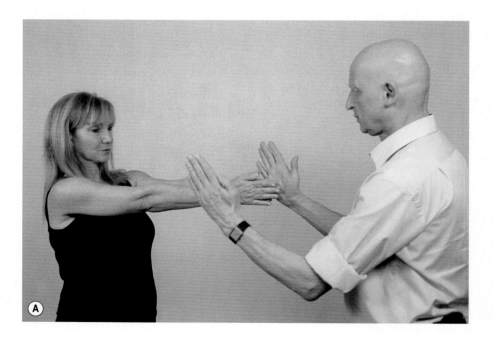

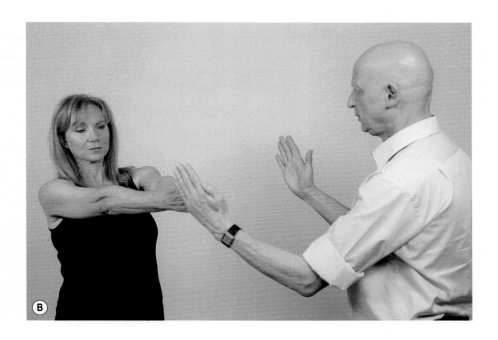

Fig. 13.65A,B: Range/free movement/flexion–extension cycles.

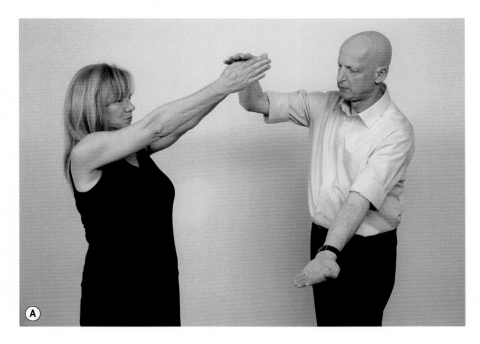

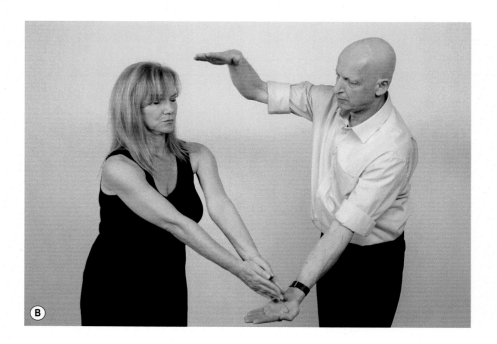

Fig. 13.66A,B: Range/free movement/complex mix of spinal movement ranges.

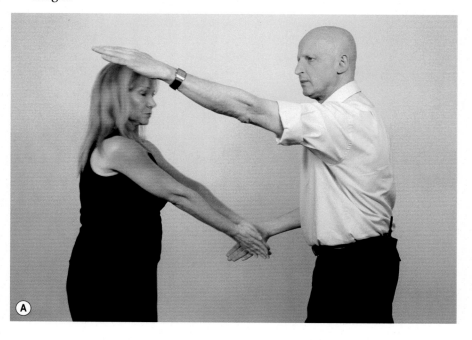

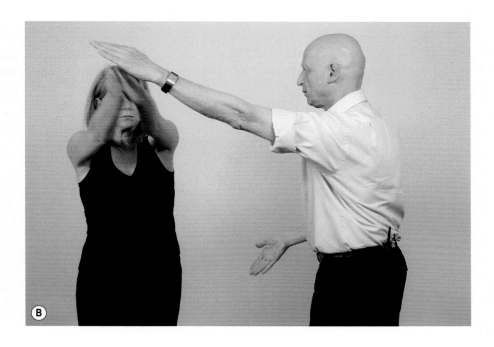

Fig. 13.67A,B: Range/free movement/primary challenge: extension/
secondary challenge: side-bending and rotation.

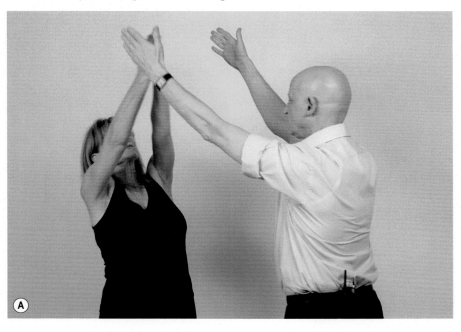

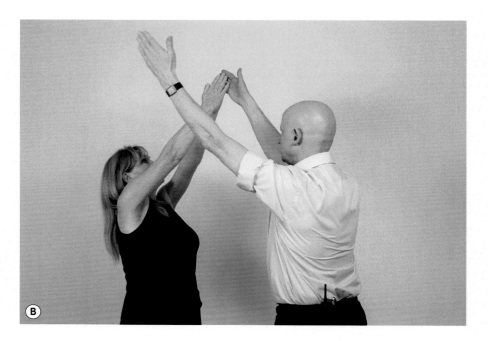

Fig. 13.68: Range/free movement/complex side-bending, flexion–extension and rotation. The patient is instructed to draw numbers on the opposite wall (0–10). As the patient's pain-free range increases the movement can progress from small- to large-amplitude numbers.

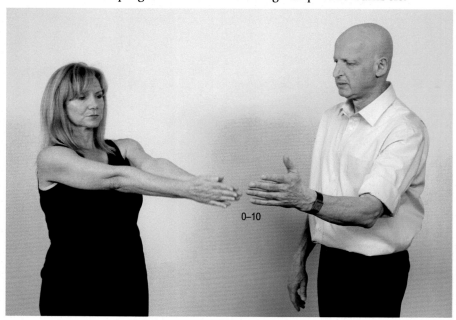

Fig. 13.69: Range/free movement/primary challenge: rotation/secondary challenge: complex side-bending and flexion–extension cycles. Instructions to patient: "Draw numbers from 0 to 10 on the opposite wall". As in Fig. 13.68, but the patient draws the number while fully rotated.

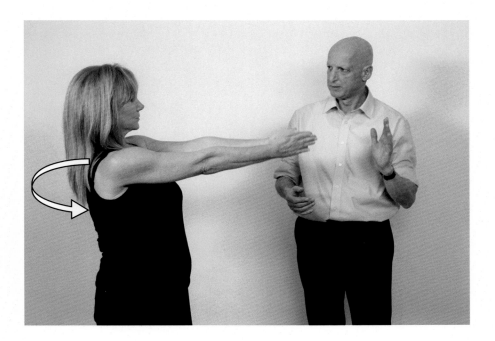

Fig. 13.70: Range/free movement/primary challenge: side-bending. As in Figs 13.68 and 13.69, the patient is instructed to reach for the therapist's hand and draw numbers on the wall to the side.

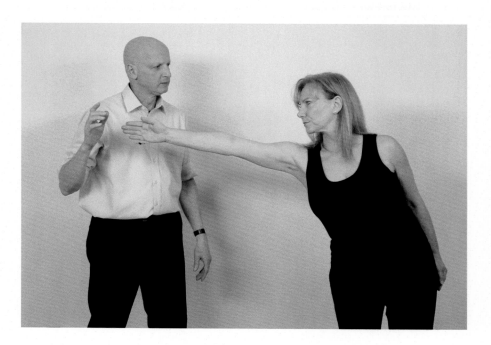

Fig. 13.71A,B: Range/free movement/different forms of life-like side-bending.

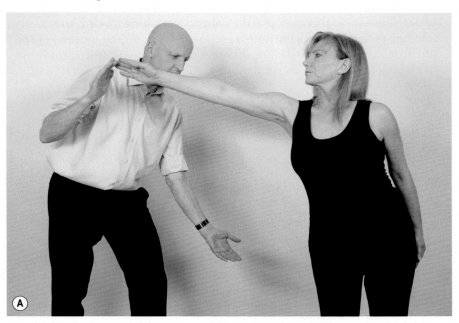

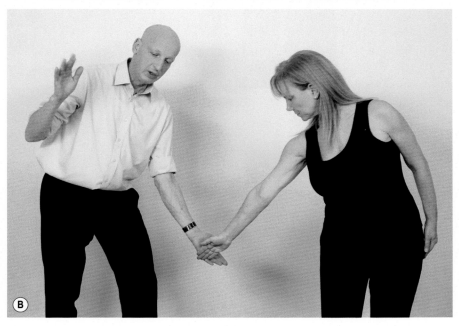

Fig. 13.72A–C: Range/free movement/rotation. Variation of trunk rotation challenge using reaching movements. Often, side-bending exercises given during rehabilitation are dissimilar to movement patterns observed during daily activities. In this example, the patient is reaching towards the therapist's hand, producing more functional side-bending movements of the trunk (this is also useful for shoulder rehabilitation). Instructions to patient: "Reach and touch my hands".

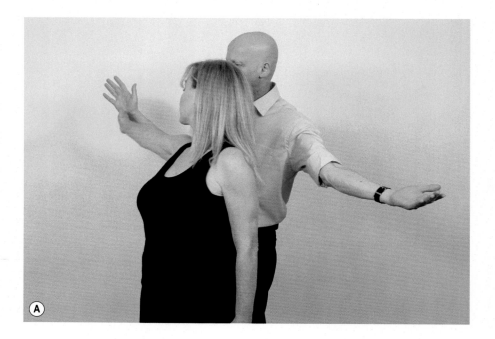

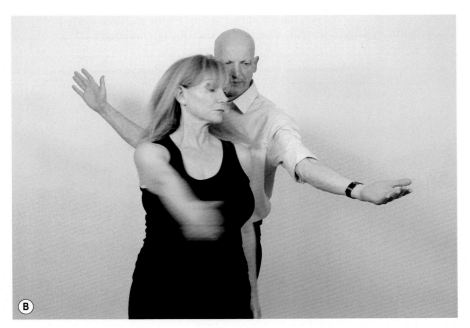

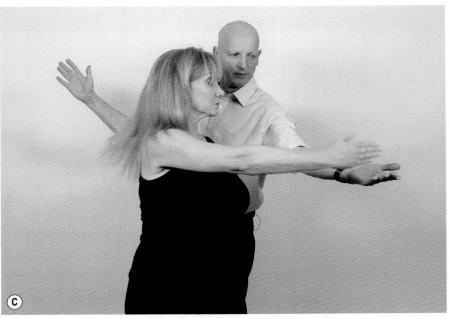

Fig. 13.73A,B: Same as challenge in Fig 13.71 but using an everyday object to highlight the functional purpose of the challenge.

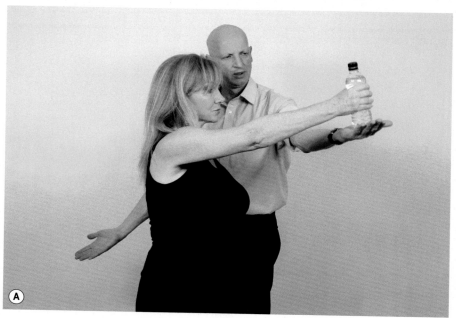

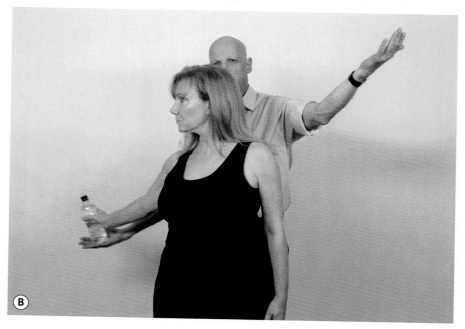

13.4.2 Seated challenges

Seated trunk challenges can be useful to localize the movement to the trunk. However, patients with low back pain may find these challenges aggravating. They should be used only in conditions where there are tissue-related ROM losses.

Fig. 13.74A,B: Range/free movement/flexion–extension cycles.
Instructions to patient: "Move the bottle from one hand to the other".

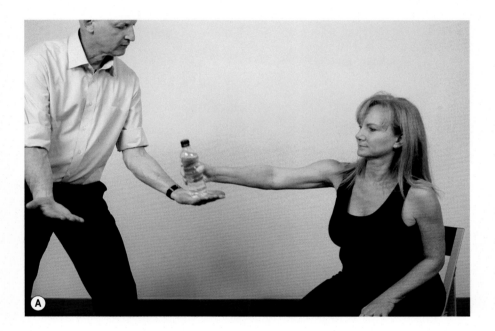

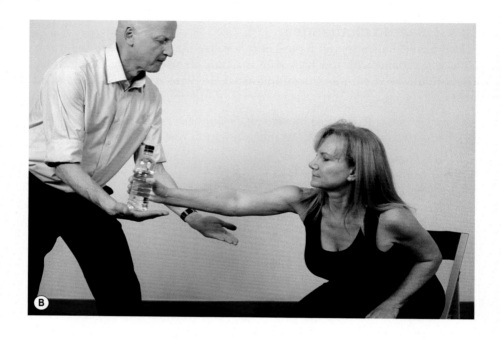

Fig. 13.75A,B: Range/free movement/rotation. Instructions to patient: "Move the bottle from one hand to the other".

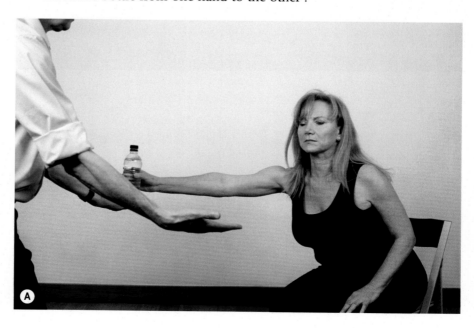

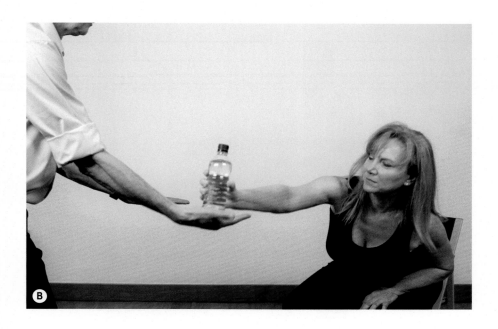

Fig. 13.76A,B: Range/free movement/side-bending. Instructions to patient: "Place the bottle from one hand to the other".

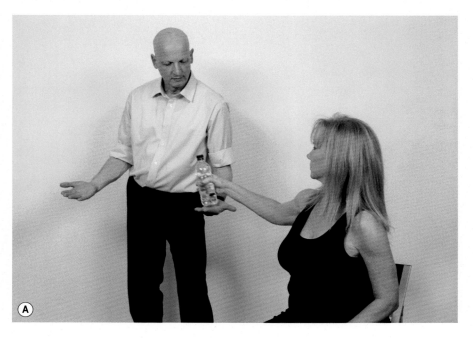

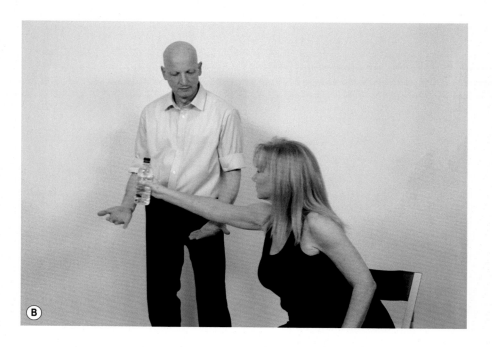

Fig. 13.77A,B: Range/free movement/mix of ranges. Instructions to patient: "Place the bottle from one hand to the other".

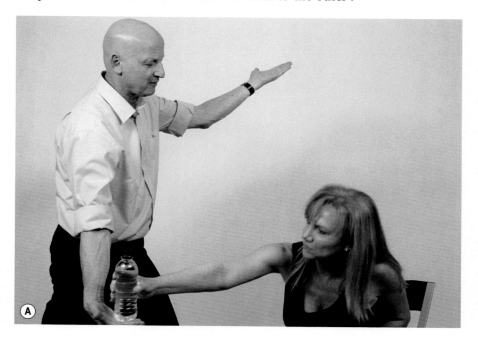

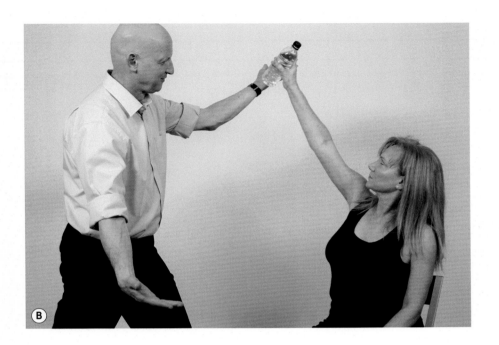

CHAPTER 14

Summary

WHAT IS THERAPEUTIC STRETCHING?

- Stretching is the behaviour a person adopts to recover, increase or maintain their range of movement (ROM)
- Therapeutic stretching is the process used to recover or improve ROM
- ROM challenges are the different techniques and methods used to achieve ROM change

WHAT MODEL IS USED FOR THERAPEUTIC STRETCHING?

- The therapeutic stretching promoted in this book uses a functional model for ROM rehabilitation
- A functional approach aims to employ the patient's own movement repertoire to facilitate ROM recovery
- It is based on the principles of recovery behaviour. It is the behaviour a person adopts to recover their functionality after injury or immobility
- The recovery behaviour contains three traits that are important for ROM recovery: specificity, overloading and repetition
- Specificity is how closely the ROM challenge resembles the affected functional movement. Overloading is the progressive increase in physical demands on the affected movement, and repetition is the overall exposure to the challenge
- ROM recovery is associated with three recuperative processes in the body: repair, adaptation and symptomatic relief; processes that encompass the tissue, neurological and psychological–behavioural dimensions
- ROM rehabilitation aims to engage the patient in behaviour that facilitates these recuperative processes
- ROM recovery is a multidimensional process intrinsic to the individual but also highly influenced by their environment. Hence, in functional

rehabilitation we aim to co-create with the patient environments that challenge their ROM losses

HOW ARE THERAPEUTIC STRETCHING TECHNIQUES CLASSIFIED?

- ROM challenges can be either functional or extra-functional
- Functional challenges are active approaches that resemble daily movement patterns. Extra-functional challenges are dissimilar to normal daily patterns
- The functional approach contains managed and assisted recovery behaviour
- In managed recovery behaviour the therapist helps the patient to develop a self-care daily programme using specificity, overloading and repetition components of the recovery behaviour
- In assisted recovery behaviour, the therapist provides physical assistance during functional tasks
- All traditional stretching methods, whether active or passive, are extra-functional

WHY DO WE NEED A FUNCTIONAL APPROACH?

- A functional approach is needed because traditional stretching approaches have been shown to be ineffective for recovering ROM in many musculoskeletal conditions
- Functional ROM challenges, including managed and assisted approaches, all contain the effective ingredients necessary for engaging the recuperative processes (repair, adaptation and modulation of symptoms)
- Extra-functional ROM challenges, including all traditional passive and active stretching approaches, provide only a few or none of the effective ingredients necessary for repair, functional adaptation and long-term management of pain

WHEN DO WE USE A FUNCTIONAL APPROACH OR TRADITIONAL STRETCHING?

- ROM rehabilitation should strive to be functional at a level that matches the individual's movement capacity
- Regressing to a lower level, below the patient's current capacity, is likely to reduce effectiveness and may prolong recovery
- If the patient is able to perform functional tasks, avoid extra-functional challenges, i.e. traditional methods

- Extra-functional challenges can be used if the patient is unable to perform functional tasks
- Extra-functional passive challenges can be used if the patient is unable to perform active movements
- A functional approach does not exclude the use of extra-functional exercise or stretching techniques

WHAT DEFINES END-RANGE?

- ROM contains active and passive components set within variable and (often) ill-defined end-ranges
- In healthy individuals active ROM is often determined by the capacity of agonist muscles to overcome antagonistic tissue tension
- Passive ROM is determined by tissue resistance. This will influence the angle at which the person will experience pain and discomfort. How far a person will stretch beyond that point will depend on their pain tolerance
- Most daily activities are performed within a small percentage of the full active ROM

WHEN IS MOVEMENT CONSIDERED FUNCTIONAL (NORMAL) OR DYSFUNCTIONAL (ABNORMAL)?

- Functional movement is the unique movement repertoire of an individual
- Functional movement contains shared activities which are universal to all and special activities which are unique to each individual
- Functional ROM is defined as the ROM required to perform functional activities effectively, efficiently and comfortably
- Dysfunctional ROM is defined as the ROM limitation that impedes the ability to perform functional movement
- Clinical-anatomical ROM ideals strive for anatomical ROM perfection
- Functional ROM is a patient-centred goal associated with recovering functionality
- Functional ROM goals are often more important than clinical ones. Most individuals judge their improvement by their ability to carry out daily activities.

WHAT CAUSES ROM LOSS?

- ROM loss in often the outcome/symptom of a condition
- Loss is often multidimensional with changes seen in the tissue, neurological and psychological dimensions

- In the tissue dimension ROM losses can be due to adaptive tissue changes and mechanical and chemical irritation
- In the neurological dimension, it can be due to loss of motor control and nociceptive processes such as sensitization
- In the psychological dimension, movement-related anxieties may also contribute to ROM loss

WHAT IS THE POTENTIAL FOR ROM RECOVERY?

- The potential for ROM recovery is dependent on the prognostic nature of the causative condition and the body's recuperative processes of repair, adaptation and modulation of symptoms
- The conditions that cause ROM loss can be classified as self-limiting, persistent or progressive
- ROM recovery is more likely in self-limiting conditions in which the recuperative processes are saved
- ROM rehabilitation will have a diminishing effect in persistent and progressive conditions, in particular if the adaptive or reparative capacity of the affected tissue is reduced, or when symptoms cannot be alleviated

WHAT HAPPENS IN ADAPTIVE ROM LOSS AND RECOVERY?

- The musculoskeletal system has the capacity to adapt to the physical environment
- Tissue adaptation is associated with *mechanotransduction*: a process by which the myocytes and fibroblasts convert mechanical signals into biological processes
- In immobilization and remobilization, adaptive processes can be seen in all musculoskeletal tissue
- Adaptive ROM loss is associated with shortening and stiffening of connective tissue, adhesion and muscle shortening and atrophy
- During ROM recovery the deleterious effects of immobilization are reversed and normalized

WHAT DRIVES ADAPTIVE RECOVERY?

- The drive for adaptation is multidimensional: it contains psychological and behavioural factors
- Adaptive processes are driven by the individual's actions within their environment

- The person's behaviour determines tissue loading and the stimulation of mechanotransduction
- ROM challenges in the form of amplified recovery behaviour, exercises and stretching can be seen as part of a physical environment that drives adaptation
- The success of ROM rehabilitation is not inherent in any single stretching approach but in the overall management

WHY IS SPECIFICITY IMPORTANT?

- Specificity is the unique motor, muscular and tissue adaptation brought about by exercise/rehabilitation
- Transfer is the measure of how the gains from the ROM challenge carry over to improve the goal task
- Transfer is more likely to occur if the training/rehabilitation resembles the goal activity, i.e. overhead reaching is improved by overhead reaching.
- Training which is dissimilar to its goals is unlikely to transfer any gains to that task, i.e. biceps curls may not be as effective in improving overhead reaching
- Many traditional stretching approaches, active or passive, are often dissimilar and lack task specificity, and as such they are unlikely to be therapeutically effective
- Task-specific rehabilitation is likely to be more effective than extra-functional/traditional stretching methods

HOW MUCH FORCE IS REQUIRED FOR STRETCHING?

- Functional ROM is maintained by the forces imposed on the body by daily activities
- Overloading is a training condition for adaptation in which physical challenges are raised above functional levels
- Underloading is the absence of sufficient forces required to maintain functional activities; it results in atrophy and adaptive ROM loss
- Forces below the overloading threshold will be ineffective at inducing long-term ROM change
- In ROM pathologies, functional activities may generate sufficient forces for adaptation
- Manual stretching approaches may fail to generate sufficient force for overloading
- Functional activities and managed recovery behaviour may provide sufficient forces for adaptive ROM recovery

CAN TISSUE LOADING BE MADE SAFE?

■ Tissue loading can be made safe by gradual introduction and amplification of forces over several weeks – graded challenge

■ During the graded challenge, all four movement parameters are incrementally amplified (force, speed, range and endurance), and there is also an incremental increase in the number of activities

■ A gradual challenge is useful for monitoring for adverse reactions, but also for reassuring the patient and the therapist that movement is safe

■ The graded challenge can be dropped back a step if an adverse reaction is encountered

HOW LONG AND HOW OFTEN SHOULD THE EXPOSURE TO STRETCHING BE?

■ ROM recovery represents a competition in adaptation between the pathological process that maintains the condition and the ROM challenge that counteracts it

■ It is estimated that, in the presence of pathology, the daily ROM challenges should be for several hours

■ Currently, there are no clear guidelines on the scheduling of traditional stretching approaches

■ In patients with ROM pathologies, traditional stretching approaches are unlikely to provide sufficient exposure for adaptation to take place

■ Only by incorporating the ROM challenge into the daily activities is there a possibility that sufficient exposure will take place

WHAT DO WE AIM TO RECOVER IN THE ACTIVE RANGE?

■ The aim of rehabilitation in the active range is to drive neuromuscular adaptation

■ The focus is on movement control and, in particular, on control of the four task parameters (force, range, speed and endurance)

■ In many musculoskeletal, pain and central nervous system conditions the control of the task parameters is attenuated

■ In functional rehabilitation the aim is to recover functional movement by amplifying the four task parameters

■ Amplification takes place while performing the affected tasks

SHOULD MOVEMENT BE FRAGMENTED OR REHABILITATED AS A WHOLE?

- The organization of movement is whole and integrated with its goals
- ROM rehabilitation should be of whole movement, goal-orientated and within a functional task
- Internal focusing strategies on specific muscles or joints turns them into the goal of movement and reduces the effectiveness of rehabilitation
- Regression to focusing on single muscles, muscle chains or joints should be the last option in any treatment

CAN PASSIVE MOVEMENT OR STRETCHING IMPROVE THE ACTIVE RANGE?

- Motor learning and functional movement and recovery are all active events
- Motor control cannot be recovered by passive challenges
- During passive techniques there is no active motor engagement
- Task-specific muscle recruitment is not being practised
- Passive stretching represents a profoundly fragmented approach that reduces the movement to the level of the muscle and the (ineffective) reflexive
- Passive approaches should only be used if the patient is unable to execute an active movement
- Active ROM should be rehabilitated with active movement

CAN TRADITIONAL ACTIVE APPROACHES IMPROVE MOTOR CONTROL AND FUNCTIONALITY?

- Muscle energy techniques and proprioceptive neuromuscular facilitation stretching as well as dynamic and ballistic stretching are all extra-functional approaches. They do not resemble "real" functional movement. As a consequence they may fail the specificity condition for adaptation
- Active extra-functional approaches are often therapist-dependent and therefore are unlikely to meet the extensive exposure needed for adaptation, particularly in the presence of an adaptive ROM pathologies
- Active extra-functional approaches promote movement fragmentation
- Active extra-functional approaches may be useful in conditions in which the patient has lost the capacity to execute a recovery behaviour or perform whole movement

IS IT POSSIBLE TO HAVE ROM LOSS WITHOUT TISSUE CHANGES?

- ROM loss can come about by increased sensitivity (sensitization) in the affected area
- Sensitization is a neurological process in which the central nervous system can change, distort or amplify the experience of pain
- ROM sensitization is a neurological process in which pain, discomfort or stiffness are experienced in normal ROMs
- In many chronic musculoskeletal conditions, ROM sensitization can be the primary cause of ROM losses; it can be present in the absence of inflammation, tissue damage or adaptive changes
- In these conditions, the patient's experience of stiffness does not reflect adaptive tissue changes; stretching is therefore ineffective for recovering ROM in conditions in which sensitization is evident

HOW DO WE DESENSITIZE ROM OR ALLEVIATE PAIN?

- Persistent ROM sensitivity may be alleviated by approaches that incorporate psychological and physical means
- Physical approaches including active and passive approaches may provide some transient pain alleviation and desensitization
- Sustained, long-term desensitization is more likely to occur by psychological and behavioural interventions that may include self-maintained exercise
- Stretching techniques are ineffective in managing acute pain
- It is unclear whether stretching is useful for alleviating chronic pain; any effect it produces is likely to be modest

STRETCH OR WAIT?

- In acute conditions, pain and sensitization have a useful protective function; improvement in pain and sensitization are often linked to overall recovery
- In acute conditions, stretching or challenging end-ranges is unlikely to be useful and may even increase the likelihood of re-injury
- During the acute phase the therapeutic focus should be on supporting recovery. Stretching is counter-indicated; it is neither beneficial nor safe
- Maintaining functionality within comfortable ranges is essential for supporting repair. Instruct the patient to maintain their daily activities as far as possible

- In chronic conditions, pain and sensitivity have no obvious protective function
- Desensitization is likely to be safe and beneficial in chronic conditions
- Overloading is likely to be safe in chronic conditions in which there are adaptive tissue changes and desensitization
- As a safety measure the ROM challenges should be introduced in a graded manner (graded challenge)

WHAT IS STRETCH TOLERANCE?

- Stretch tolerance is a "learned dissociation" between the experience of stretching pain and injury
- ROM gains following long-term regular stretching may be associated with stretch tolerance but also with adaptive tissue changes
- A stretch-tolerance model fails to explain ROM loss or recovery in conditions in which adaptive tissue changes have taken place
- This model is important in conditions in which ROM losses are associated with sensitization (Ch. 9)
- A stretch-tolerance model fails to elucidate the mechanisms underlying long-term gain of flexibility by regular stretch training
- The stretch-tolerance model has no training implications for healthy individuals who aim to increase their agility
- Adaptive–behavioural models are far more important for agility training and managing recovery in conditions where ROM losses are associated with adaptive tissue changes

WHAT IS THE CONTRIBUTION OF PSYCHOLOGICAL FACTORS TO ROM LOSS AND RECOVERY?

- ROM loss can be maintained by avoidance behaviour due to fear of pain and re-injury
- Anxieties about movement can be due to misinformation, a learned association between pain and movement or to anxiety traits that predate the condition
- The alleviation of movement-related anxieties can be in the cognitive and behavioural spheres
- In the cognitive sphere, reassurance can be given by providing information about the condition, in particular positive messages that increase the individual's belief in their ability to care for and control their condition
- Reassurance in the behavioural dimension can include a gradual reintroduction of activities which are important for the patient

HOW CAN WE IMPROVE ADHERENCE?

- Keep the patient positively informed
- Identify goals that are important to the patient
- Make the challenges readily available
- Provide ongoing support and feedback
- Keep it simple
- Make it fun

WHAT'S NOT IN THIS BOOK?

- 50 different techniques to stretch the hamstrings or any other muscle in the body
- Detailed anatomy of every muscle in the body
- Long lists of joint assessments
- Dry biomechanics
- Muscle chains
- Muscle-by-muscle rehabilitation
- Movement fragmentation
- Specific tissue mobilization
- Fascial network and stretching
- Evidence-based protocols
- Clinical certainty

FINALLY

- Use what the patient already knows for the rehabilitation. It is effective and economical
- Construct the ROM challenge as part of the habitual daily movement repertoire
- Many daily activities can be exaggerated to challenge ROM losses at home. This should be the emphasis of the management
- No two patients or conditions are alike, but they share management similarities
- Be creative-devise the managment with the patient
- The ultimate message is – promote self-care, whenever possible

Index

Page numbers followed by "f" indicate figures, "t" indicate tables, and "b" indicate boxes.

Printed in the United States
By Bookmasters